ASTHMA

& HAY FEVER

A SELF-HELP GUIDE

COMBINING ORTHODOX AND COMPLEMENTARY APPROACHES TO HEALTH

HEADWAY HEALTHWISE

ASTHMA & HAY FEVER

A SELF-HELP GUIDE
COMBINING ORTHODOX AND COMPLEMENTARY APPROACHES TO HEALTH

HASNAIN WALJI & DR ANDREA KINGSTON

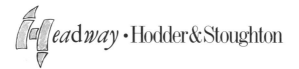

Headway · Hodder & Stoughton

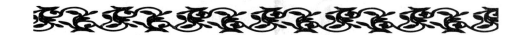

Cataloguing in Publication Data is available from the British Library

ISBN 0 340 60558 8

First published 1994
Impression number 10 9 8 7 6 5 4 3 2 1
Year   1998 1997 1996 1994 1994

Printed in Great Britain for Hodder & Stoughton Educational, a division of Hodder Headline Plc, 338 Euston Road, London NW1 3BH by Page Bros (Norwich) Ltd.

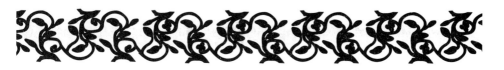

CONTENTS

Foreword To The Series 8

Foreword To The Book 9

Preface 11

1 Overview: Oh No! It's Spring Again 15

2 Orthodox Medicine: What Can Your GP Offer? 25

3 Nutrition: Let Food Be Your Medicine 41

4 Herbs: Nature's Pharmacy 54

5 Homoeopathy: Like Cures Like 63

6 Anthroposophical Medicine: An Extension To Conventional
  Practice 74

7 Aromatherapy: Not Just An Exotic Treatment 82

8 Other Techniques: Breathing And Stress Control 93

    Osteopathy

    Chiropractic

    Reflexology

    Acupuncture

    Acupressure

9 Conclusion 113

Glossary Of Terms 116

Index 120

The Natural Medicines Society 122

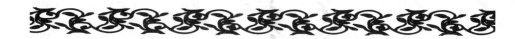

*This book is dedicated to the seekers of health
and to those who help them find it.*

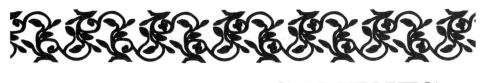

ACKNOWLEDGEMENTS

I should like to express my gratitude to Dr Andrea Kingston for her valuable input, not just from from a GP's point of view, but also for the enlightened way she dealt with a number of apparent contradictions between orthodox medicine and complementary therapies; to nutritionist Angela Dowden for offering many pertinent suggestions; to Sato Liu of the Natural Medicines Society for her assistance in providing contacts and arranging interviews with practitioners; and to my agent Susan Mears for her encouragement and practical help.

   This book could not possibly have been written without the co-operation of the following practitioners who have so willingly endured my interruptions: acupuncture – John Hicks and Peter Mole; aromatherapy – Christine Wildwood; naturopathy – Jan De Vries; chiropractic – Jatinder Benepal; herbal medicine and Alexander Technique – Rick Brennan; homoeopathy – Michael Thompson; anthroposophical medicine – Dr Morris Orange; and osteopathy – Jonathon Parson. A practitioner who must be singled out for special acknowledgement is homoeopath Beth MacEoin, for her so very prompt and painstaking review of the chapter on homoeopathy.

   I must thank my daughter Sukaina for giving her time during vacation from university for wading through research papers and books and extracting relevant information. Last but not least, I wish to thank my wife Latifa whose gentle care and concern, not to mention long hours typing the manuscript, enabled me to complete this book.

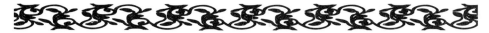

Foreword To The Series
from the Natural Medicines Society

When we visit our doctor's surgery and are given a diagnosis, we often receive a prescription at the same time. More people than ever are now aware that there may be complementary treatments available and would like to explore the possibilities, but do not know which kind of treatment would be most useful for their problem.

There are books on just about every treatment available, but few which start from this standpoint: the patient interested in knowing the options for treating their particular condition – which treatment is available or useful, what the treatment involves, or what to expect when consulting the practitioner.

The Headway Healthwise series will provide the answers for those wishing to consider what treatment is available, once the doctor has diagnosed their condition. Each book will cover both the orthodox and complementary approaches. Although patients are naturally most interested in relieving their immediate symptoms, the books show how complementary treatment goes much deeper; underlying causes are explored and the patient is treated as a whole.

It is important to stress that it is not the intention of this series to replace the expertise of the doctors and practitioners, nor to encourage self-treatment, but to show the options available to the patient.

As the consumer charity working for freedom of choice in medicine, the Natural Medicines Society welcomes the Headway Healthwise series. Although the Natural Medicines Society does not recommend people who are taking prescribed orthodox medicines to stop doing so, our aim is to introduce them to complementary forms of treatment. We believe the orthodox system of medicine is often best used as a last, not first, resort when other, gentler, methods fail or are inappropriate.

Giving patients the information to make their choice is the purpose of this series. With the increasing use of complementary medicine within the NHS, knowing the complementary options is vital both to the patients and to their doctors in the search for better health care.

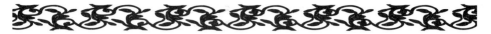

Foreword To The Book

In recent years, asthma – particularly in children – has grown to the proportions of an epidemic in western countries. This has been a rapid and bewildering development and, like the rise in chronic illness generally, it casts a long shadow over the future.

I can remember, as a schoolboy in the early 1960s, being the only pupil in my year – and one of the very few in a large school – to suffer from the condition. To be asthmatic then was to be something of a rarity. Today, in schoolrooms round the country, children line up their inhalers at the start of the day's lessons and pick them up when they leave. Something drastic has happened in thirty years.

On the one hand, modern medicine may have all but eliminated infectious childhood diseases, as a recent report claimed. On the other, the increase in chronic illness in both children and adults is alarming. Modern drugs can ameliorate many of the symptoms of asthma. I will always be grateful for the freedom that my first inhaler, which I was given when I was fifteen, introduced into my life. If nothing else, it enabled me to start attending school regularly for the first time, to obtain good A-level results in consequence, and to go on to a successful university career that laid the basis for most of my later work.

But inhalers, steroids and other drugs do not offer a cure, and recent studies have even suggested that 'the regular use of asthma "puffers", such as Ventolin, can make the condition worse, rather than better' (*The Guardian*, October 1993, citing a report in *The Lancet*). Many of these drugs can and do save lives and are appropriate therapy in numerous instances; but their long-term impact on the health of patients is only one of many counter-indications that make a quest for safer measures a matter of the utmost importance.

It is here that the potential of alternative medicines is immediately evident. Not only have serious alternatives to conventional medicine risen enormously in popularity in recent years, but scientific study of their effectiveness has advanced by leaps and bounds and has opened up new vistas on the future direction of health care and sickness management, particularly for chronic conditions.

Instead of the costly and frequently unsuccessful hunts for 'cures'

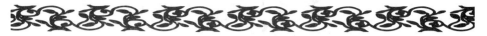

that have characterised orthodox medical research in the last century, we are likely to see in coming years a broader, more holistic approach to illness, an approach that will enable us to see people as individuals rather than bearers of disease labels like 'asthmatic' or 'a hay fever victim'. And we may see a growing emphasis on prevention and the control of environmental factors in place of the current concern with patching and mending.

Since beginning homoeopathic treatment, I have seen my own asthma improve for the first time in almost forty years. My use of Ventolin has dropped dramatically, even in cold, damp weather, and I have increasingly long spells when I do not use it at all. I firmly expect to throw my inhaler away in due course, and I am certain that I would have done so a long time ago had I come to homoeopathy earlier, ideally as a child. But at least a new generation of children, more prone to asthma though they may be, will have far greater opportunities for receiving alternative treatments that may reduce or eliminate their illness and free them from life-long dependence on suppressive and potentially harmful drugs.

Asthma & Hay Fever is designed to introduce readers still fresh to such matters to the range of possibilities available from alternative and complementary therapies. It shows the extent and limitations of orthodox treatments and describes, in detail, what sufferers may expect when they visit a homoeopath, acupuncturist, herbalist or whatever. There is helpful advice on general preventive measures and on nutrition, together with a survey of elementary, self-help measures – always on the understanding that treatment of difficult, chronic conditions is almost certain to be beyond the capabilities of the beginner and that prolonged, serious case management by a trained professional is essential if lasting improvement is to be hoped for.

Just buying *Asthma & Hay Fever* is a step in the right direction. It is not a book about miracle cures or overnight recoveries, and your asthma or your hay fever will not be gone next week. What this book does show is a rational way forward. It places your child firmly on a road that, travelled carefully and in the company of experienced guides, may lead to marked improvement in your and their health and, should all go well, to permanent recovery.

Denis MacEoin MA PhD
Author (Daniel Easterman) and Council Member of the
Natural Medicines Society

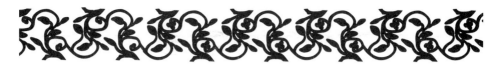

PREFACE

Headway Healthwise is a concise new series which takes the original approach of looking at common ailments and describing how they may be treated using complementary therapies. The aim of the series is not to replace the orthodox medical approach but to give readers an overview of how they may be helped by consulting complementary practitioners.

Once a condition has been diagnosed by a GP, those wishing to avail themselves of other forms of treatment will find this book particularly useful. The intention of this series is not to recommend that people who are taking prescribed orthodox medicines should stop taking these; it is to introduce them to alternative and complementary forms of treatment which may enable them to reduce the number of orthodox prescriptions they take and, in some cases, to obviate the need for orthodox prescriptions altogether.

We have attempted to present the information in a style that is clear and easy to read. The central approach is to look at asthma and hay fever from different perspectives by providing you with descriptions of several complementary therapies. While cautioning against self-medication, the book has been written to encourage you to take charge of your own health by making an informed choice of therapy.

An overview of asthma and hay fever and the kind of treatment to expect from your GP is covered in the first two chapters. The third chapter deals with such factors as lifestyle, diet and nutrition in the management of asthma and hay fever. Later chapters look at complementary approaches to the subject.

The one common factor that underpins all the alternative or complementary therapeutic techniques described in this book is the belief in the healing power of the body. Practitioners recognise that the body possesses an inherent ability to cure itself. This gives a clear message to the patient of his role in the healing process – that of the mind willing the body to heal itself.

At first sight this may appear to challenge the approach of orthodox medicine, in which the therapeutic objective is to cure the diseased part of the body. The patient has no role to play except

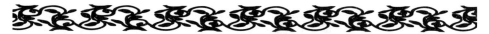

dutifully to take the medicine. The concept of a white-coated god who possesses the magic pill to cure is the result of fear combined with a lack of understanding of the nature of disease and, more so, that of health.

This book is an attempt to dispel the myths and to bring about a greater understanding of the issues relating to health and healing, which go beyond the realms of simple anatomy and biology. The recognition that orthodox medicine and complementary therapies need not be mutually exclusive can go a long way towards promoting the integrated medicine of the twenty-first century.

Hasnain Walji
Milton Keynes
November, 1993

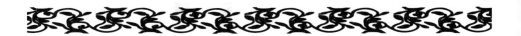

Note: Any information given in this book is not intended to be taken as a replacement for medical advice. Any person with a condition requiring medical attention should consult a medical professional.

OVERVIEW: OH NO! IT'S SPRING AGAIN!

It's spring. The birds are singing and the sun is shining. The trees are in full bloom. A gentle breeze wafts through the undulating meadows and rustles the grass. Bliss! Or is it? Your eyes are smarting, your nose streams and you sneeze – ceaselessly. Your throat is sore, your chest is tight and you cannot sleep at night.

Almost four million people in Britain await the summer with trepidation. Their bags bulge with tablets, inhalers and other medications, and they have to drive with their car windows shut. For them it is the season of misery; they are the vast army of people who suffer from hay fever.

It was Charles Blackeley in 1873 (a sufferer himself) who first discovered that pollen was one cause of hay fever. It is said that he sent kites high into the air with sticky plates to collect pollen. He tried sniffing pollen at various times throughout the year, and actually rubbed samples on his skin to produce the symptoms of hay fever.

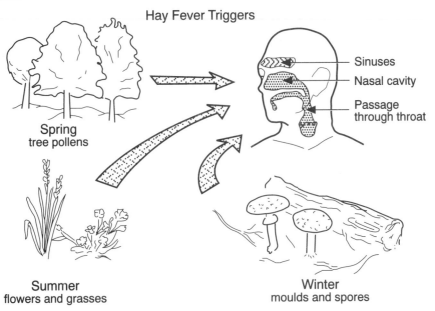

Hay Fever Triggers

Spring
tree pollens

Sinuses

Nasal cavity

Passage
through throat

Summer
flowers and grasses

Winter
moulds and spores

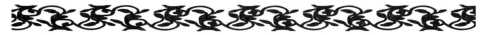

Pollen is released as plants reach the peak of their growth – it is nature's way of ensuring their survival. Interestingly, it is not the most colourful flowers that cause most trouble but the less showy ones. This is because the plants with the most colourful flowers rely on insects to transfer pollen. The less showy plants have much finer pollen spores to enable the spores to be carried on the wind, and these are much more likely to penetrate the lining of the air passages. Pollen grains are rich in proteins, and when they enter the body through the air passages, they may cause an allergic reaction. This is known as *pollinosis.*

Similar reactions,however, can also be precipitated (brought on) by other substances This condition, virtually identical to pollinosis, is called *allergic rhinitis.* When we breathe we inhale many different kinds of airborne particles. These can include particles of feathers, fur, fabrics, moulds, food, human skin scales, hair, fibre from carpets, clothes and upholstery, and the droppings of the *Dermatophagoides pterynissinus,* the house dust mite. Viewed under a microscope it is a fearsome-looking creature, but actually it is its excrement that causes the most trouble.

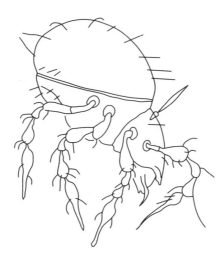

The house mite

In most cases, the nose is able to filter large particles before they reach our lungs. But if the membrane is weak for any reason, or if we are obliged to breathe through our mouths because of a blocked nose or strenuous physical activity, then particles enter our bodies and can give rise to a number of allergic reactions. Sometimes occurring in the same person, hay fever and asthma are common

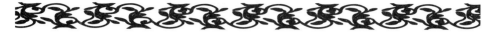

conditions, which affect more than 15 per cent of the population.

Hay fever is a real nuisance as it can interfere with work, school and play for weeks on end, but it is asthma which causes most anxiety. This is quite rightly so, since it can be a life-threatening condition in a minority of people, if inadequately treated.

Both conditions have become more common in the last 20 years. Theories for this increase include better diagnosis by doctors, greater atmospheric pollution and our changing eating habits.

What Causes Hay Fever?

Very simply, hay fever is the result of the body's overreaction to pollens and other airborne particles. The human body has an in-built system of defence against disease and has the ability to heal itself. Called the *immune system*, it is the body's own fighting force. It is spurred into action as soon as it encounters intruders in the form of bacteria, viruses and other foreign matter. It is when the immune system overreacts and starts attacking harmless foreign substances that an allergic condition develops. Hay fever is a good example of the result of an overreaction, as pollen is, in itself, innocuous.

Excessive amounts of a substance called *histamine* are released by the body, producing itching, swelling, a runny nose, watery eyes and a sore throat. Histamine is a chemical which helps maintain normal brain function, but in excess causes inflammation of the mucous membranes *(mucosa)* lining the eyes, nose and air passages, giving rise to the uncomfortable symptoms of hay fever.

What Causes An Allergy?

As already mentioned, an allergy is caused by the body's tendency to overreact to substances entering the body which would normally be well tolerated. Any substance that causes an allergic reaction is called an *allergen*. In the case of hay fever, the allergen is pollen.

Most allergens are protein particles which the immune system perceives as foreign invaders. The immune system can learn how to identify the special protein of the invader substance and make a chemical antidote which will attack that specific protein. The chemical antidote is called an *antibody*, and the foreign protein it is created to immobilise is called an *antigen*. There are many different types of antibodies, collectively known as *immunoglobulins*. The medical term for the antibody specifically involved in hay fever is called *immunoglobulin E (IgE)*.

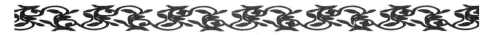

The principal combatants of the body's defensive system are found in our bloodstream. Called *lymphocytes*, these cells patrol the body in search of foreign invaders. There are different roles for different combatants: the T-cells, regulate the immune system and have the ability to decide whether to attack or to withdraw and, when necessary, engage in direct combat with invaders; the B-lymphocytes secrete antibodies and have the ability to remember their targets so that they can supply the antibody much faster in the event of a subsequent attack. As long as the immune system is working efficiently, disease can be kept at bay. (This topic will be dealt with in greater detail in Chapter 3.)

In the case of hay fever, when the membranes lining our airways in the nose, sinuses and lungs are penetrated by pollen or other airborne particles, the body's fighting militia is spurred into action. The result is the production of IgE, which sensitises the *mast cells*. Mast cells are large white blood cells which are found in abundance in the mucosa. These mast cells then become 'leaky', and release chemicals, such as histamine and leukotrines, which set up an inflammatory reaction in the mucosa. The result is that the mucosa becomes swollen and produces an increased amount of mucus. This is called *sensitisation* (see Chapter 2).

Asthma

The expression 'As natural as breathing' reveals just how much we take breathing for granted. Yet when asthma strikes, breathing is far from natural and we have to fight for every breath and, in extreme cases, for our very life.

The word 'asthma' comes from a Greek word meaning 'panting'. The Greek physician, Hippocrates (460–370 BC), recommended that asthmatics should avoid shouting and anger! But it was not until the sixteenth century that the ailment was correctly understood. In the late seventeenth century, in his *Treatise of the Asthma*, Sir John Floyer observed that 'all Asthmatics being angry or sad, do fall into Fits oftener than they are cheerful', thus reflecting the emotional aspects of the ailment. Among physicians in the nineteenth and early twentieth century, asthma was regarded as a trivial condition. Oliver Holmes, an American physician, called it 'a slight ailment which prolongs longevity'!

Even today, the definition of asthma continues to cause controversy. A useful working description is 'a condition with

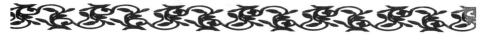

recurrent attacks of breathlessness accompanied by wheezing and varying in severity from hour to hour and day to day, caused by the narrowing of the airways in the lungs'. It is generally accepted that 1 in 20 of the overall population in the UK suffers from it, and that the prevalence in children can be as high as 1 in 10.

The three most characteristic symptoms of asthma are a cough, wheezing and shortness of breath, especially on physical exertion. The symptoms can vary in severity and duration, depending on the individual. In some cases, there may be a painful tightness in the chest and a great deal of effort required to empty the lungs, so much so that the muscles in the neck and the abdomen are seen as rigid bands as they try to aid the chest muscles.

As the air escapes from the lungs through the narrowed tubes, a wheezing sound is produced. Breathing is further impaired as the large amounts of frothy mucus produced during an attack may lead to coughing and even choking.

Common Forms of Asthma

Asthma is a long-term illness. The more common form of asthma is correctly termed *bronchial asthma* to distinguish it from *cardiac asthma,* a condition associated with wheezing caused by heart failure.

Bronchial asthma can often be related to hay fever or eczema, or hereditary factors. In this type of asthma, there are usually well-defined factors that trigger attacks. In addition to pollens, house dust, animal fur, infections, exercise, and even emotions, can bring on an asthma attack. It is with this form of asthma that hay fever is more likely to be connected.

Asthma can also be brought on by an infection of the airways. This type of asthma tends to recur constantly and is more severe, as the narrowing of the airways tends to be less easily reversible. In addition, it can vary in severity and then sometimes disappear for years, only to reappear without any obvious reason.

If you are a parent of an asthmatic child (there are 150,000 schoolchildren in the UK who suffer from asthma) you maybe anxious to know if your child will grow out of the condition. Various studies on this subject indicate that three-quarters of the children grow out of their asthma by the age of 10. However there is no guarantee that it will stay away – in a third of cases, asthma returns after the age of 20.

It would appear that the inclination to asthma in adults is greater

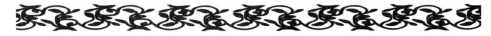

for those who were asthmatic in their childhood. Commonsense measures, such as minimising contact with the allergens that spark off attacks, coupled with diet and lifestyle measures, reduce the likelihood of the disease recurring.

An Asthma Attack

Our lungs operate as an exchange mechanism. Oxygen from the air we inhale into the lungs enters the bloodstream to be pumped around the body. Carbon dioxide 'waste' crosses back from the bloodstream into the lungs and leaves the body when we exhale.

During an attack of asthma, this function is impaired, as breathing requires the lungs to be free of obstruction and an asthma attack is a result of obstruction in the lungs caused by the narrowing of the airways .

The Narrowing Of The Airways

To understand how narrowing occurs, we must first look at the structure of the airways and how air passes between the nasal passage and the lungs.

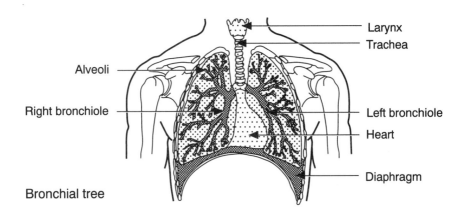

The airways are made up of the nasal passage, the throat (upper part of the *pharynx*), the voice box (the *larynx*), the windpipe (the *trachea*), the main air passages (the *bronchi*) and smaller air passages (the *bronchioles*). The windpipe contains tough and elastic tissue called *cartilage*, which makes the windpipe wall 'stiff' and less likely to narrow.

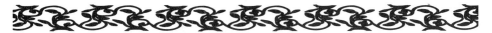

Both the trachea and the bronchi are lined with a mucous membrane which provides moisture and traps dust and foreign bodies. All the airways are covered by an *epithelium*, which is like a thin skin. On top of this skin there are minute hairs called *cilla*, which constantly sweep mucus upwards in the direction of the throat. Underneath the epithelium lie smooth muscle and glands that secrete mucus. Called *bronchial glands*, they have little tubes opening into the surface of the airways through which they pour out mucus secretions.

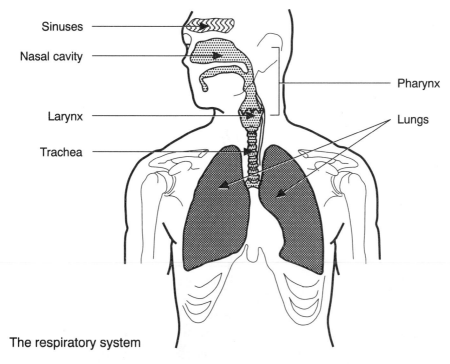

The respiratory system

In asthma patients, the glands tend to produce mucus which is extremely sticky, and this contributes to the narrowing of the airways. In severe cases, the sticky mucus can virtually block most of the air passages, which can be fatal. But it is the hypersensitivity of the smooth muscle of the trachea and the bronchi to various stimuli (like pollen, dust, exercise and infection) that results in an asthma attack. The nerve endings in the smooth muscle are stimulated by the dust or pollen and send a signal to the brain. The brain responds by 'telling' the smooth muscle to contract and narrow the airways.

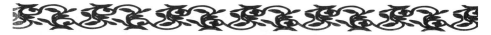

Triggers Of Asthma And Hay Fever

The most obvious triggers are those that bring on the symptoms of a runny nose and streaming eyes in cases of hay fever, or wheezing and coughing in asthma. Some sufferers are able to recognise immediately the factors that will bring on an attack. Obviously, if the triggers are things such as animal fur, then these can be easily avoided. Triggers such as pollen or house dust mites are impossible to avoid, though contact can be minimised by, for example, changing linen more often, staying away from open fields during the spring, wearing a mask when mowing the lawn. Other triggers, such as food, are more difficult to detect and, in any case, there is a great deal of controversy in the medical profession about this subject. The general consensus among conventional practitioners is that food allergies in themselves are quite unusual, but that many substances that we take in, such as additives and, in particular, colourings, can cause symptoms in the gut without an allergic reaction. This is called *food intolerance* as opposed to an allergy.

Environmental Triggers

House Dust Mites
- most common allergen responding to tests
- found virtually everywhere, but a warm, humid atmosphere suits them best
- generally found in household dust, but mainly in soft furnishings, dust traps, fluffy toys, bedding and pillows
- feed on human skin scales
- too small to be seen with the naked eye, too big to be inhaled
- their droppings are small enough to enter the airways
- sufferers get better in an environment free of mites, but this is not really practical

Pollens
- released at various times of the year, but most abundant in the spring and summer
- trees, such as silver birch, grasses, such as Bermuda grass, Timothy grass and cocksfoot, and plants, such as mugwort, ragweed and oil seed rape, are particularly troublesome in spring
- mould spores growing on grain and rotting vegetation in the autumn
- *Aspergillus*, a fungus that grows on rotting vegetation, can be particularly harmful to some asthmatics

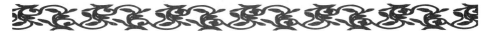

Animals
- cats are more likely to cause problems from allergens in their hair, skin, urine and saliva
- dogs, rabbits, horses and rodents can all be sources of allergens

Pollution
- cigarette smoke is by far the most common form of pollution
- sulphur dioxide in factory smoke
- exhaust fumes and smog

The Weather
- sudden changes in temperature and humidity, particularly for asthma patients
- an increase in fungal spores due to humidity
- an increase in the number of airborne pollen grains and other pollutants

Exercise
- asthma connected with the drying and cooling of the airways in the lungs
- exercising in a warm, moist environment is least likely to trigger an asthma attack
- an indoor swimming pool is more suitable than an outdoor one

Food
- food allergy is a controversial issue among doctors, and many prefer the term 'food intolerance'
- the reaction is not really an allergy involving antibody response, but a reaction to a particular chemical
- foods connected with asthma are dairy products, nuts, colourings and fizzy drinks

Infections
- infections of the upper respiratory tract
- colds, flu and sore throats

Drugs
- *propranolol* – a drug used to reduce blood pressure
- nonsteroidal anti-inflammatory drugs used for arthritis
- aspirin

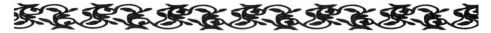

Is there A 'Cure'?

There is a general consensus of opinion among the orthodox medical profession that there is no cure for asthma and hay fever. The response, therefore, has been to produce various drugs, such as anti-histamines (that neutralise the histamine) or steroids (used for their anti-inflammatory properties), to enable suffers to control the symptoms. Other procedures, such as desensitisation and vaccinations, have been devised to confront the symptoms. For asthma, in particular, bronchodilator drugs that increase the diameter of the airways for a short period are popular interventions (see Chapter 2). Complementary therapists, however, look at the root cause to treat the condition.

While most drugs are effective in giving short-term relief and are absolutely essential in severe attacks, there are a number of lifestyle and nutritional measures that can go a long way to minimising the impact of these ailments (see Chapter 3). In view of the fact that both hay fever and asthma are caused by the malfunctioning of the immune system, a positive plan of action can be invaluable in ensuring that the body's natural ability to heal itself is operating at maximum efficiency. The management of hay fever and asthma, as with any other ailment for that matter, requires a change in our perception that health is not just absence of disease, but a positive sense of well-being.

In the following chapters, we shall look at the signs, symptoms and causes of hay fever and asthma in some detail, as well as the different therapeutic options available in the management of these ailments.

2

ORTHODOX MEDICINE: WHAT CAN YOUR GP OFFER?

The first person you are most likely to turn to for advice and treatment for asthma and hay fever is your family doctor. Fortunately, nearly all GPs' surgeries are now well equipped to deal with asthma and allergy-related emergencies. Many lend out equipment, such as nebulisers (instruments for applying a liquid in the form of a fine spray), for sufferers during asthma attacks. The number of health promotion clinics held at surgeries is now on the increase, and you will find that the practice nurse may run an asthma or allergy clinic to monitor progress and to help with the many inhaler devices available.

Most doctors now appreciate how important it is to ensure that the patient understands how a treatment works. With such allergy-related conditions as asthma and hay fever, it is all the more important that there is a joint effort between the GP/nurse and the patient in managing the condition. This not only helps the patient to detect what triggers the problem, but also assists in planning avoidance where possible. Above all, it enables the sufferer to take responsibility for his or her health, to understand the condition and thereby to take prompt action in an emergency.

Let us look at hay fever first, as it is a less serious condition than asthma.

How Do You Know You Have Hay Fever?

Many people diagnose hay fever quite easily, especially if it occurs at the same time each year and lasts the same number of weeks. Probabiy a large percentage of sufferers do not even bother to visit their GP and either put up with the symptoms, or treat themselves with over-the-counter medications available from the local pharmacy.

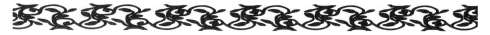

In children, however, hay fever is sometimes difficult to recognise. Parents, and even doctors, sometimes dismiss the symptoms as a series of colds and viral infections. The condition is rare in children under the age of 3, and still uncommon in those under 5. Young children with hay fever often develop a typical face. Constant rubbing of the nose or eyes, mouth breathing or snoring can all give clues. The nose may develop a permanent crease across the bridge from constantly being rubbed upwards by the palm of the hand. This is called the 'allergic salute'.

An *atopic* child (that is, one with an inherited predisposition to various allergic conditions) may also develop dark rings under the eyes known as 'allergic shiners'. This is due to the sluggish flow of blood around the blocked nose.

There is a possibility that a child suffering from hay fever may develop asthma at the same time: about 5 per cent of the children do. So it is important, if you are worried, to consult your GP. Usually, he or she will try out a treatment and monitor the progress of your child over a number of weeks.

Finding An Allergy In Order To Avoid It

Some people have an allergic response to just one substance. An example of this would be pollen, say, from a particular species of flower. The symptoms of a runny nose, sore eyes and sneezing may start quite abruptly and the cause is then obvious. Many adults, however, are allergic to more than one substance. It could be trees, pollen, grasses or moulds. They may have a delayed response to an allergen of up to 24 hours. Most atopic children have multiple allergies.

Allergies in children may change and develop as the children get older and they are exposed to new substances. The problem is compounded when hay fever has already started in children and the lining of the nose then becomes more sensitive to other irritants, such as cigarette smoke or perfume. To a large extent, these irritants can be avoided until treatment gets under way. It is well worth keeping a diary of symptoms and activities to try and pinpoint a specific allergen.

One way of testing for allergies is the *skin test*. This may be performed either at a special allergy clinic or under the supervision of a skin specialist. Solutions of a variety of pollens, moulds, etc, are placed on the skin which is then pricked to allow entry under the

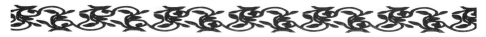

surface. Redness and swelling will indicate an allergic reaction. Only a minority of people are actually referred by their GP for specialist investigation, and only a small number of these are helped by the results.

For most people, avoiding allergens, such as pollen, is virtually impossible. Pollens are easily spread in the air, even inside the home. Some sufferers may choose to take holidays by the sea where pollen counts are generally lower. But for most people medical treatment becomes necessary to allow them to carry on with their normal, everyday lives.

Types Of Treatments

If you have hay fever you will want an effective treatment that is not likely to cause any side-effects. Though modern medicine has yet to come up with a 'cure', certain procedures and drugs have been devised to relieve the symptoms.

Antihistamines

These are the most commonly prescribed medications in the treatment of hay fever. There are many different types of tablets and syrups, including some long-acting, once-daily preparations which are available without prescription. They act by 'blocking' the action of histamine. A major drawback of many of the earlier antihistamine preparations was that they caused drowsiness. The newer preparations, for example, terfenadine and astemizole, generally do not. However, some individuals may still become drowsy and should not drive or operate machinery while they are taking them. The longer-acting preparations are not suitable for young children. Most GPs will prescribe a drug called prochlorperazine (trade name: Piriton) which is given three times daily.

Anti-allergy Drugs

Developed in the late 1960s, sodium chromoglycate (trade names: Opticrom and Rynacrom) is a drug that acts on the mucous membrane, the lining of the nose and the eyes. It prevents calcium from entering the cell thus inhibiting the release of histamine. In other words, it stabilises the cells present in the membrane and stops them reacting to allergens. However, it can do nothing to stop the action of histamine once it has been released. Such drugs need

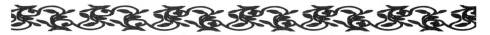

to be taken throughout the hay fever season whether symptoms are present or not. Available in the form of eyedrops and nasal sprays, sodium chromoglycate is effective only when taken regularly, and may have to be used four or more times daily.

Steroids

Because of their anti-inflammatory properties, steroids are effective for severe forms of hay fever and asthma. They suppress the immune response and give effective short-term relief. Their long-term use is controversial, as the effects of suppressing the immune system may impair the immune system itself. Steroids given for long periods of time may also lead to unpleasant side-effects.

Local steroids can be administered by the use of aerosol sprays, and are now often prescribed for adults and children alike. Beclomethasone (trade name: Beconase) and flunisolide (trade name: Syntaris) have been shown to be more effective than sodium chromoglycate preparations and have almost no immediate side-effects. Administered twice daily, they are effective after two days and this usually continues to build up over a number of weeks. They are available either in an aqueous spray, which most people find comfortable to use, or in a dry aerosol spray. Doctors recommend these sprays particularly because they prevent nasal polyps (small growths) which are sometimes associated with hay fever and allergy.

Oral steroids, such as prednisolone or Betnelan, provide quick relief within a few hours for people who suffer severe symptoms. Doctors give them in courses over two or three weeks, or intermittently when the pollen count is high. There is very little risk of side-effects and no tailing off the dose is necessary. They are particularly useful for important occasions, such as interviews, weddings and examinations, and, once working, will give the sufferer confidence that relief is possible while other treatments are started.

Injected steroids are the last resort for people with very severe symptoms who will not take other forms of medication, or who find all other treatments ineffective. One example is the drug Kenalog. The steroid injection is given deep into the muscle of the buttock. It usually starts to act within 48 hours, and is effective for several weeks in most people and remains in the body for several months. The effects of injected steroids cannot be reversed once given. They may interfere with the body's own hormones in women and cause

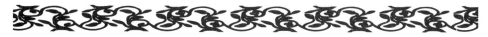

irregular periods. Prolonged use in hay fever is rare, and it can cause the wasting of the muscle around the injection site.

This form of treatment is quite popular for, once tried, many people find it 'addictive'! So discuss it thoroughly with your GP first. Remember, also, if you are planning a pregnancy, that long-acting steroids may harm the developing child.

Decongestants

Fast-acting decongestants applied directly into the nose, available without prescription from your pharmacist, give quick relief from the nasal congestion associated with hay fever. However, their action is short lived and somewhat variable. Overuse decreases their effectiveness still further, and long-term use can damage the sensitive lining of the nose.

Desensitisation

This is a process whereby small purified amounts of the allergens are injected into the individual to try to make the immune system 'tolerant' of the substance. The procedure can cause some local reaction and, even worse, a whole-body allergic reaction, producing severe shock. A few people have died as a result of this reaction.

A small minority of individuals may benefit, however, particularly those who are sensitive to only one substance, usually a pollen. In any case, you would be well advised to have the desensitisation procedure done under the supervision of a specialist and in a hospital where resuscitation equipment is available. Although a life-saving measure for those who react severely to bee stings, for most hay fever sufferers this method is not very effective. Since its introduction in the 1970s, it has largely fallen out of favour with the medical profession.

Asthma – A Serious Condition

Asthma is a condition that affects young and old alike. At one time, it was considered a disease of the well born and sensitive. There are more than two million sufferers in Britain today and, despite better diagnosis and treatment, there are still around 2,000 deaths a year of which 50 are children. An inquiry into the death rate has shown that a significant number of deaths are thought to be caused by the patient or the GP not recognising the severity of the problem.

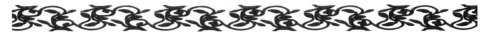

Inadequate treatment, especially failure to use steroids early enough, are believed to account for half of the deaths. While many children will grow out of their asthma, it should still be considered a chronic and unpredictable condition.

Several recent studies have looked at people's understanding of asthma. There is an overwhelming consensus among these studies that those who understand their asthma well are more likely to take their medication regularly and are less likely to suffer a serious attack. In countries where over-the-counter medications, including inhalers, are available, people visit their doctors less frequently. A recent study of people who bought their medications over the counter showed that they have very poorly controlled asthma, underscoring the need for consultation and monitoring by a medical professional.

A Special Problem For Children

Asthma can begin in infancy, often following a lung infection or flu. Around 11 per cent of 17 year olds have had at least one episode of wheezing in their lives and, by the age of 10, 20 per cent will have had some signs.

Isolated episodes of wheezing in response to, say, a viral infection, do not constitute asthma. Recurrent attacks, often accompanied by other atopic conditions, will confirm a diagnosis. Very young babies can develop wheezing since their airways are highly sensitive to trigger factors. If a baby has recurrent episodes, he or she will be more likely to develop asthma later on.

In young babies other conditions need to be excluded, such as cystic fibrosis, congenital heart and lung disease and tracheo-bronchmalacia.

Treatment for wheezing in babies under a year old is generally unsatisfactory. The reason for this is that bronchodilators, drugs that have the effect of 'opening up' the narrowed airways, cannot work on young babies. This is because bronchodilators work on the smooth muscle around the bronchial tree, and there is very little of this muscle in children until 12 to 15 months of age.

In the majority of children, however, diagnosing asthma is relatively easy. There may well be a family history of asthma, eczema or hay fever. If a child has one parent with asthma, there is a 25 per cent chance that he or she will be affected; with two parents afflicted with asthma, this rises to 40 per cent.

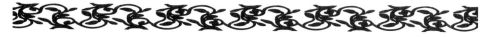

In most cases, there is an allergic cause of the problem. Studies have shown that a high proportion of asthmatic children, around 80 per cent, show an allergic response to the house dust mite. There is a large variety of other allergens. Animal fur, feathers, grasses and the pollens that trigger hay fever can all be equally implicated in asthma.

Pets are easy to identify as a source of allergen. All members of the cat family are more likely to cause symptoms when their hair and dander (tiny particles of skin) are inhaled. Circus performers, vets and zoo attendants are known to be affected by lions, tigers and jaguars. Hamsters, guinea pigs, rats and mice can also be responsible for an allergic reaction.

Trigger Factors

Things that cause the sensitive airways of the asthmatic to react, but do not actually cause an allergic response, are called *trigger factors* (see also Chapter 1).

Emotions

At one time it was thought that if you had asthma you were 'unduly sensitive', and the condition was generally labelled as a psychosomatic disorder, possibly resulting from childhood conflict within the family. Now we know that it is very much a physical condition and that asthmatics are no more 'sensitive' than the rest of the population, and that while emotions such as crying and laughing, or even being anxious, can trigger asthma, they are not actually causes. Of course, severe asthma can be disturbing and can cause distress, not only to the sufferer, but also to other members of the family. Sibling rivalry can be generated as it is easy for brothers and sisters to feel that the asthmatic child receives an unfair share of parental attention. Some children do get very adept at invoking symptoms when it suits them and it is, understandably, hard for the parents not to give in to their demands.

Exercise

This is another common trigger factor where up to 80 per cent of children can have their asthma induced if they exercise briskly enough. This is probably due in part to the drying of the airways. It was therefore thought that exercise was bad for asthmatic children.

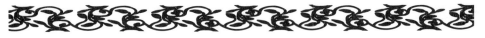

However, experts now recommend that moderate and controlled exercise can actually be of benefit to many. In 1982, an international symposium on the asthmatic child in play and sport made a number of recommendations:

- control of exercise intensity and duration
- prolonged warm-up periods
- intervals during training
- avoidance of exercise when the air is dry and cold
- increased aerobic fitness

Swimming is perhaps the best form of exercise. Attacks of asthma have been found to be less severe afterwards.

The Weather

Sensitive airways are a feature of the illness, and sudden changes in the weather can trigger attacks. Temperate, humid conditions seem to suit asthmatics better than cold, dry air. Of course, the pollen count during sunny weather is higher, resulting in a greater incidence of attacks. Damp, late summer and autumn days can also trigger attacks, as the level of moulds in the atmosphere increases. Holidays by the sea or in the mountains, which provide a change of environment, are helpful.

Pollution

The most obvious source of pollution is cigarette smoke. A recent study has clearly shown that children in smoking households are more likely to develop asthma. The smoke may act as a sensitiser. Its role as an irritant is acknowledged, and we know that children in smoking households are more likely to develop chest infections.

Nocturnal Asthma

It is not uncommon for children to have trouble with asthma at night, either with a persistent cough or with an increase in their wheezing. At one time, it was thought that the body's own steroids were at a lower level during this time, though subsequent studies have discounted this. Sensitivity to the house dust mite is a potential trigger, as is an allergy to feathers. Pets should be removed where possible. However, some children still wheeze more at night, and it is likely that there are a number of other factors contributing, as yet

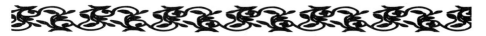

unknown. If your child has problems at night, it may indicate that the overall control of asthma is poor and needs careful review, and you would be well advised to consult your GP.

It is best to report mild and transient wheezy breathing, occuring for the first time in a child, to the doctor.

Diagnosis of Asthma

Although some children may present very suddenly with an episode of severe wheezing, this is relatively unusual. It is much more common to have wheezing (with an upper respiratory infection) or persistent coughing at night or after exercise.

Your GP will usually ask questions about your family and possible trigger factors. Since the wheezing may be intermittent, there may be nothing to find when the child is examined. An exercise test will usually sort out the matter if exercise is thought to be a trigger. The child might be asked to run about for at least 6 minutes, and your doctor will listen again to hear if any wheezing has developed. A very important part of the examination is measuring the peak respiratory flow. This is to assess the degree of obstruction due to the narrowing of the airways. Blowing into a peak flow meter allows the rate at which air is expelled from the lungs to be measured. The rate depends on sex, age and height. Peak flow increases with age to a peak at around 35 years old, and then slowly starts to decline. A peak flow of 15 per cent or more below normal, in combination with a history of predisposition to asthma, will very strongly indicate a diagnosis of asthma. The peak flow meter is now available on prescription (it is mentioned further on page 35).

Investigation

In most children and many adults, no special investigations are needed because the diagnosis is obvious. In children who seem to be severely disabled, and in most children who have attacks that take them to hospital, further investigation is inevitable, usually in terms of a chest X-ray and sometimes blood tests to see if there is a response to a particular allergen. The average child who presents with mild to moderate wheezing does not usually need any special tests.

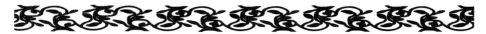

Severity

Attacks can vary in severity. The medical profession has classified the forms of asthma according to their degree of severity. It is useful to know these classifications because they predict the outcome and, to a large extent, the treatment that is required for children.

Infrequent And Episodic

This is the mildest form, which is commonest in 4 to 6 year-olds and usually follows an upper respiratory infection. Seventy-five per cent of children have asthma in this category.

Frequent Episodic

This is when the child has more than six episodes a year. The triggers are most commonly viruses and exercise. Allergies also play a large part. Twenty per cent of children have this moderate form of asthma.

Chronic Persistent

This is when there is a persistent airflow obstruction. The children are markedly atopic, that is, have multiple allergies, and may suffer from hay fever and eczema. This more severe form of asthma represents 5 per cent of children affected. It is these children who may have significant absences from school and who may suffer from retardation of their growth (this is discussed in more detail on page 37).

Outlook For Children With Asthma

This is very much dependent on the severity of the condition. For those children who have infrequent and episodic asthma, about three-quarters are entirely free from wheezing by the age of 14 years. Of chronic persistent asthmatics, only 20 per cent will be free from asthma by this age.

Unfortunately, asthma may be a recurrent condition, and though children may be free for several years, it may recur in adulthood for reasons that are not clear. This makes the knowledge of trigger factors doubly important.

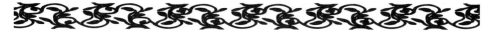

Asthma In Adults

Diagnosis can be difficult, as wheezing may occur in other conditions, such as heart failure or chronic bronchitis and emphysema (otherwise known as *chronic obstructive airways disease*). A number of chemicals can also cause asthma in the working environment. One example is isocyanates, used in the manufacture of plastics and in paint spraying. These chemicals can also sensitise the lungs to other trigger factors. There may also have been a history of 'bronchitis' in childhood which, on further questioning, turns out to be undiagnosed asthma.

There can be further complications with adults in that the condition may coexist with other problems. Someone with chronic obstructive airways disease, for example, may develop asthma as well.

There is often a reluctance for adults to admit to this, especially older people who may remember friends and relatives who suffered quite badly before the newer treatments and inhalers were available. Older people often need more convincing about the need to comply with treatment than children.

The Peak Flow Meter In Diagnosis And Monitoring

This basic piece of equipment measures the fastest rate at which air can be expelled from the lungs (a simple measurement of the diameter of the airways). The rate varies with age, sex and height, and is at its greatest around 35 years of age and then slowly declines. Peak flow meters have been available on prescription since 1990. Reduction of at least 15 per cent in a peak flow reading is indicative of airflow obstruction and asthma, but asthmatics' airways may vary much more widely by up to 50 per cent.

If there is some doubt about diagnosis, the meter can be very useful, especially for those children who are coughing at night but are symptom-free during the day.

The meter helps asthmatics to recognise the onset of an attack. Some sufferers are not aware that a severe attack is coming on until a very late stage. It is also useful for monitoring the progress of treatment, which can be a great encouragement in getting adults and children to take their medication regularly. The technique of blowing hard into the mouthpiece comes easily with practice.

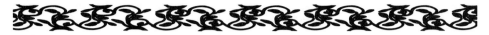

Medical Treatment

There are drugs which give immediate relief from wheezing *(bronchodilators)*, and there are those which are used for the longer-term treatment and prevention of asthma.

Beta-adrenergic Bronchodilators

These are the commonest forms of treatment (for example, salmeterol and terbutaline). They are related to the hormone adrenaline, but are most specific in acting on the smooth muscle around the airways, causing it to relax and open up. They have a more specific effect on the lungs than adrenaline, but they may still cause the heart to beat faster. Mostly used as inhalers, they can also be given in syrup to young children, by nebuliser or, in emergencies, by injection from a doctor.

Salmeterol is a new beta-adrenergic bronchodilator that has been used over the last three years in adults, but has only recently been licensed for use in children. It is different from the other beta-adrenergic bronchodilators in that it has a much longer duration of action, at least 12 hours. Two recent studies have shown it to be particularly good for exercise-induced symptoms in children. It is also very useful in the management of night-time symptoms in adults.

Salbutamol (trade name: Volmax), given in slow-release tablet form, can be useful for night-time symptoms if patients cannot or will not use a steroid inhaler.

Anticholinergics

Available under such trade names as Oxivent and Atrovent, anticholinergics are drugs which act by blocking signals to the main nerve supply to the lungs, the vagus nerve. They can be administered by inhaler, nebuliser or syrup. Some very young children may benefit from them where other drugs fail, and they are sometimes given in conjunction with other bronchodilators.

Xanthine Derivatives

Xanthine derivatives have an effect of dilating the bronchules. Under names such as theophylline, aminophylline, (trade name: Uniphyllin) xanthine derivative drugs are used as tablets or, less

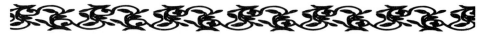

commonly, in injection, and are related to caffeine. They may also be given to children in the form of a syrup, although they can cause stomach irritation, nausea and vomitting. Xanthine derivatives have an effect of dilating the bronchules.

Preventive Treatment For Asthma

Such treatment is really only necessary for anybody who has more than six episodes of wheezing per year. It should certainly be considered for anyone who has been ill enough to need hospital admission. Corticosteroids have been included here, although they are sometimes used for acute episodes of asthma. They are effective after several hours.

Anti-allergy Drugs

Examples of these include sodium cromoglycate and nedocromil sodium.

While adults may benefit from this drug when used in the nose and eyes, only a small proportion are helped when it is inhaled into the lungs. It may also be used in nebuliser form. It is a useful drug for children who are known to have a specific allergy, and in those who have exercise-induced asthma. It is best taken 15 minutes before exercise. Like all preventive medicines, it has to be taken regularly to be of use, and a course should probably continue for a minimum of six months. It has some anti-inflammatory activity on the bronchial tree, but it is now thought that the action of inhaled steroids is much more effective in reducing inflammation in the long term, and it is likely that sodium cromoglycate will be used less in the future by those who have severe asthma.

Corticosteroids

These drugs are now the mainstay of treatment for anyone who has moderate or severe asthma, but they still cause a great deal of worry for parents of sufferers because of fears of long-term side-effects. Adults, too, have worries about becoming addicted to this type of medication.

We now know that doses beyond 400 mcg a day for inhaled steroids will not inhibit growth in children. Above this, there is some suggestion that growth may be mildly delayed. The same applies to children who need oral steroids frequently. However, there is now

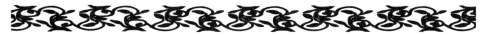

good evidence that these children catch up when the steroids are reduced, and attain their final expected height. It should be remembered that chronic severe asthma in itself can cause retardation of growth.

Most people do not need to take oral steroids but can keep in control of their asthma by regular inhalations of one or another preparation, either using one of the inhalers or, during an acute attack, via a nebuliser. A short course of oral steroids, for example, prednisolone, taken in tablet form over a week or two can be life saving and is likely to prevent a hospital admission.

Ketotifen

Taken in tablet form, this drug is an antihistamine which also has some anti-allergic properties. It is probably helpful in a few people, but it can cause drowsiness and is now used less frequently.

Experimental Drugs

Very recent tests have suggested that certain drugs used in cancer and organ transplantation may be helpful. Methotrexate, a drug used in leukaemia and other cancers, has been tried in low dosage with good effects in some asthmatics. Cyclosporin, a drug used in transplants, has also shown promise. However, both these drugs can cause severe side-effects and there is no guarantee that they will ever be used for asthma because of this.

Desensitisation

In asthma treatment, desensitisation has largely fallen out of favour for the same reasons as discussed earlier in the chapter. Certain patients may benefit, but these are generally the ones who are only allergic to one substance. Most people benefit much more from the usual inhaler treatment.

Which Inhaler?

Most adults manage very well with a standard inhaler – a pressurised canister with a mouthpiece. Children, however, are not always able to co-ordinate this, and breath-activated devices, such as a spinhaler or autoinhaler, may be helpful. Space is allowed for devices to be attached to the mouthpiece to enable the drug to be inhaled more slowly.

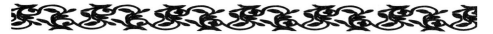

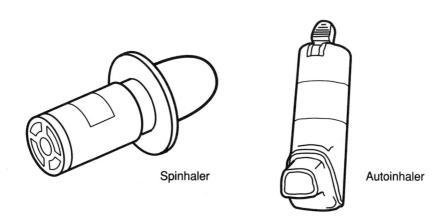

Spinhaler   Autoinhaler

Adults who are unable to co-ordinate or who are disabled and cannot go on to a canister may find it easier to use breath-activated devices as well. Dry powder inhalers, which are very compact, are popular with older children as they can easily be carried in the pocket.

Nebulisers

These are commonly used for acute asthma, and some adults and children with severe problems have their own.

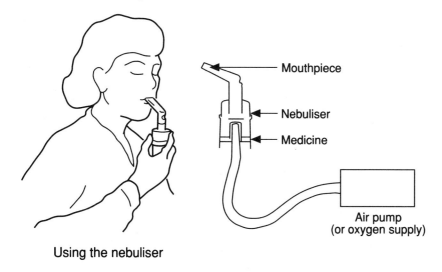

Mouthpiece

Nebuliser

Medicine

Air pump
(or oxygen supply)

Using the nebuliser

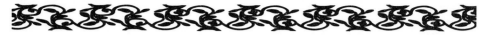

It is wise to consult your GP before buying a nebuliser. For most asthmatics, they are unnecessary and are best used for those who are unable to cope with an inhaler, and for young children. They give a high dose of the drug concerned and, when used under medical supervision, can often abort an attack and prevent a hospital admission.

Acute Attacks

Those unfortunate asthmatics who are severely ill with attacks will probably be in regular contact with their own doctors. Some will have nebulisers to use at home, and many will carry a course of oral steroids to start at the first sign of an acute attack.

It is imperative for these patients that they have good preventative treatment, usually in the form of inhaled corticosteroids, as well as bronchodilators. Most people with severe asthma should be taking regular peak flow readings so that they are aware of when their peak flow is dropping down and they can start oral steroids or seek help before they develop severe symptoms.

3

NUTRITION: LET FOOD BE YOUR MEDICINE

Eating and drinking habits can affect the incidence of hay fever and asthma. It is important to be aware of this, since this is the one area over which you have the greatest control.

You should be aiming for a wholefood diet that eliminates chemical additives and other known food allergens, such as wheat and milk. Such a diet removes a number of asthma and hay fever attack stimuli and provides a wide range of vital nutrients.

However, it is not enough to avoid foods that trigger attacks. We also need to eliminate the toxins and accumulated poisons which prevent the immune system from working at optimum efficiency. A long-term trial on 25 asthmatic patients put on a vegan diet showed that they improved significantly when the most common food allergens were eliminated. The diet excluded all meat, fish, eggs and dairy products, as well as ordinary tea, coffee, chocolate, sugar and salt. The patients were given vegetables, such as lettuce, carrots, onions, celery, cabbage, cauliflower, broccoli, nettles, cucumber, radishes and various beans and pulses. Grains were restricted, as were citrus fruits. Fruits consumed freely were blueberries, cloudberries, raspberries, strawberries, blackcurrants, gooseberries, pears and plums. Seventy-one per cent responded within four months, and over a period of one year it was found that 92 per cent showed a significant improvement in their condition.

Such a diet also helps to reduce the body's production of leukotrienes. Derived from a fatty acid called *arachidonic acid* found exclusively in animal products, leukotrines, are much more potent stimulators of bronchial constriction than is histamine.

Foods that help to replenish our defensive arsenal are also vital. They should contain main nutrients which promote a healthy immune system – vitamin A and beta carotene, vitamins C and E, and the minerals selenium and zinc.

As a general rule, keep to a low-fat, high-fibre diet which is adequate in all the vitamins and minerals, and is low in refined sugar. It should contain alkaline foods, such as fresh fruits (except

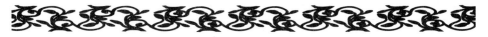

bananas, which are too starchy) and vegetables. Sprouts from seeds and grains are particularly valuable. Try to cut down on meat (particularly pork and beef) as it is acid forming. If you must have meat, then go for chicken or, better still, fish.

Catarrh is common in asthma and hay fever. To reduce it, limit your intake of cereals (even wholegrain), and avoid most dairy products. Although catarrh is formed more readily when dairy foods are taken, natural yoghurt may actually help to inhibit histamine production.

The suggestion that milk should be avoided inevitably raises eyebrows, since it is acknowledged to be a valuable source of proteins, fats and minerals, especially calcium. But some people cannot digest it because they do not have sufficient of the enzyme *lactase* which breaks down the lactose in cow's milk. This condition is called an *intolerance*. Sometimes infants who are weaned on to cow's milk at an early age develop antibodies which give rise to a milk allergy. Milk intolerance or milk allergy both promote the formation of excessive catarrh. Soya milk may be a more suitable alternative, as it is rich in protein.

It may help to avoid eating foods high in protein and carbohydrates (starch and sugar) at the same meal. Mixing the two results in the protein being only partly digested. These proteins are toxic and some may contribute to the production of histamine. Dr Hay, of who devised the 'Hay Diet', maintained that certain classes of foods are not compatible. If eaten together, they are inadequately digested and can cause a wide variety of digestive problems.

Caffeine can suppress the immune system, so all caffeine-containing beverages and drinks should also be avoided.

And, believe it or not, sugar is the cause of *hypoglycaemia*, or low blood sugar. Refined sugar is rapidly absorbed by the body. The blood sugar level rises and triggers the pancreas to secrete the hormone insulin. Insulin causes sugar to be absorbed into the body tissue. Normally, the sugar is quickly used up, but the insulin remains circulating in the body extracting what sugar is left in the blood. This creates a craving for more sugar and a vicious cycle is started. As a result, the pancreas becomes oversensitive and produces too much insulin which further results in the reduction of energy levels. This in turn undermines the immune system. Most sugar substitutes and artificial sweeteners are of little benefit as they are made from chemicals which can irritate certain tissues in the body and create more toxins.

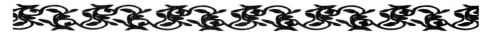

Artificial preservatives and dyes are also involved in asthma. It is essential to eliminate common colouring agents, such as azo dyes (tartrazine, sunset yellow and amaranth), and preservatives, such as sodium benzoate, sulphur dioxide and 4-hydroxybenzoate esters.

Nutrition – The Mainstay

Most orthodox and complementary practitioners will tell you that underlying all disease is the breakdown of the body's natural functions. Poor nutrition is one of the primary causes of breakdown.

Hippocrates, the father of medicine, recognised this 2,000 years ago. Yet his words, 'Let food be your medicine, and your medicine be your food', seem to have been forgotten by modern medicine.

Of course, there is no doubt that our current sophisticated knowledge of the disease process has led to the production of specific drugs to counteract or neutralise substances, such as histamine. But these drugs are of only short-term benefit. They may help to relieve the symptoms, but they do not prevent them from recurring. A return to basics, to food as medicine, is what is really needed.

It is only just emerging that changes in lifestyle and eating habits during the last one hundred years have heaped an untold burden on our bodies. We are now less able to fight disease. Indeed, we appear to suffer more often from disease than our predecessors! The body, through its immune system, has an amazing capacity to deal with the viruses, bacteria and other organisms that are an integral part of our lives. However, lack of nutrients can weaken the immune system and impair its function. If this is understood, then the role of nutrition in the prevention of disease becomes clear.

Foods To Avoid And To Increase

Avoid
- acid-forming foods
- most dairy products: cow's milk, cheese, cream, butter
- meat, especially pork and beef
- coffee, tea and drinks containing caffeine
- alcoholic beverages

Increase
- alkaline-forming foods
- fruits and vegetables

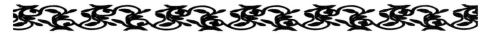

- fruit juices
- live or natural yoghurt
- herb teas

The Structure Of The Immune System

Our immune system is the body's main line of defence against both minor and major illnesses. As soon as the immune system encounters an organism that it perceives as foreign, certain cells in the body fight the organism to get rid of it. The system is so sophisticated that it can actually 'remember' the foreign organism, and is able to respond to it more quickly the next time it is encountered. This is called *acquired immunity.*

Vaccination is a good example of one way we can acquire immunity. A small amount of treated or dead organism is introduced into the body by injecting a vaccine. As the organism is already treated or dead, there is no danger of acquiring the disease. However, as soon as the body's defence force encounters it, it is put on red alert, fights it and makes antibodies to it. It will also remember how to get rid of it should it meet a similar organism in the future. So, if you were to become infected with an active live organism of the same kind, say of cholera, your immune system would be able to respond to it before the foreign organism had a chance to cause disease. All the information is stored in the *thymus gland,* the body's 'computer'. It instructs the body's defence force when to commence attack and, equally, when not to attack in the case of harmless foreign organisms.

As long as the immune system is healthy, it can fend off the onslaught of disease. But it can be compromised by poor diet, environmental pollution, stress and even the natural process of ageing, with serious consequences.

Sometimes when the system malfunctions, it becomes overactive and starts attacking harmless foreign substances. Hay fever is a classic example. Normally, pollen is harmless, and yet the immune system starts to attack pollen particles. The cells involved in allergic response come out in full force, releasing histamine and resulting in the symptoms of hay fever.

At times the immune system goes horribly wrong and actually starts attacking the body's own cells, for example in rheumatoid arthritis. Problems also arise in organ transplants because the immune system programmed to reject a foreign tissue, begins to

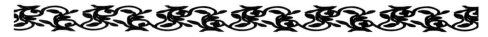

attack the new heart or kidney.

You can see how important it is to keep the immune system in a state of balance. However, the problem for the immune system in this late twentieth century is that while the human body is remarkably adaptable in its quest for survival, it needs time to change. Unfortunately, the pace of change in the environment has overtaken the body's natural ability to offer a timely response. The immune system is overworked and does not always know how to respond to the array of new enemies that confront it. Environmental pollution, the depletion of the ozone layer, pesticides and CFCs have all contributed in upsetting our finely tuned immune system. The result is that many of us live with recurring health problems – colds, flu, chronic fatigue and other diseases, including hay fever and asthma.

Furthermore, if the system cannot eliminate and detoxify a foreign organism, the body has to store it somewhere. The liver, bones, and even the brain, become the storehouses for this sometimes dangerous waste. The effects of these toxins, together with the imbalance of nutrients in our food, increases our vulnerability to disease.

Why Does Our Immune System Become Weak?

Oxygen is necessary to sustain life but, paradoxically, is also responsible for weakening our immune system. All living things that use oxygen produce *free radicals*. Free radicals are the cause of rusting iron, hardened rubber and wrinkled skin. When cells use oxygen, they produce a small proportion of unstable molecules that lack an electron (molecules are stable only when they are electronically even). These unstable oxygen molecules are free radicals. Created every minute we are alive, they are largely held in check by the body's own army of antioxidants, and as long as they are kept under control we remain healthy. However, if we begin to make more free radicals than we need (and they do serve a useful function), there is a risk of damage to the immune system and of developing chronic diseases.

Unchecked free radicals are thought to be the major cause of mutations and cancers, memory loss and senility, autoimmune diseases, ageing and wrinkles. The polyunsaturated fats that make up the body's cell walls are particularly sensitive to free radical

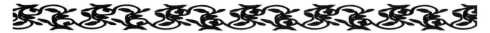

attack. They become rancid (oxidised) and are structurally damaged.

Environmental Factors

As well as the body's normal production of free radicals, there are other outside factors that can add to our free radical burden:

- excessive exposure to X-rays
- radioactive contamination
- pesticides, industrial solvents, CFCs and other pollutants

Because free radicals can be hazardous to human health, it is important to neutralise them before they do any damage.

Protection From Free Radicals

Protection from free radicals comes from antioxidants. An antioxidant is a substance that can protect foods from oxidation (going rancid) – especially fats and oils. It does this by preventing oxygen from combining with other substances and damaging cells.

The nutrients that are commonly thought of as our first line of defence against free radical attack are vitamins A, C and E, beta carotene, and the minerals zinc and selenium. (Some amino acids also have a part to play in fighting excess free radicals.) Vitamins and minerals cannot be produced by the body itself, and must come from the diet.

Vitamins, Minerals And Other Micronutrients

The statement that 'We are overfed but undernourished', makes sense once we understand why, despite having all the food we want, many of us still do not take in all the essential nutrients we need.

Our diets abound in proteins, carbohydrates and fats. These are called *macronutrients* and form the bulk of the food we eat. Vitamins and minerals, although essential, are only required in minute quantities, and so they are called *micronutrients*. Macronutrients provide energy. Micronutrients (which neither contain calories nor provide energy themselves) allow energy to be released. In fact, vitamins and minerals are a part of the structure of *enzymes* (organic catalysts that facilitate the complex biological processes to take

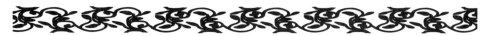

place). Disease can develop if these micronutrients are consistently missing from our daily diet.

Micronutrients are delicate and can easily be destroyed or depleted by a whole host of factors. Modern farming methods have depleted the minerals in soil. The use of pesticides together with food processing technology have further reduced the levels of these essential nutrients in our food. A deficiency of certain nutrients means that other nutrients cannot be absorbed, and the digestive functions are disturbed. As far as asthma and hay fever are concerned, the body needs higher than normal levels of certain nutrients to counter the effects of inflammation and the overreaction of the immune system.

As mentioned above, certain vitamins and minerals also function as antioxidants. By eating wholefoods that are rich in micronutrients, we can increase our intake of these antioxidants. The World Health Organisation has recently recommended a daily intake of 400 g (approximately 1 lb) of fruit and vegetables (to include beans and pulses) to keep us healthy. However, this is not always possible or practical and vitamin supplements can help.

Vitamin C

This is perhaps one of the most important nutrients for asthma and hay fever sufferers. As an antioxidant, it aids the immune system; as a natural antihistamine, it alleviates the allergic symptoms of asthma and hay fever; and as an antipollutant, it helps to eliminate toxic substances from the body.

Vitamin C (also known as *ascorbate*) is also responsible for tissue repair, the formation of antibodies and the stimulation of the white blood cells, as well as for the formation of the corticosteroid hormones in the adrenal glands.

It is is probably the most researched antioxidant substance. It is soluble in water and provides antioxidant protection for the watery compartments of our cells, tissues and organs. Our bodies cannot make vitamin C, so we are dependent upon food sources for this vital nutrient. It is worth knowing that bioflavonoids sometimes occur alongside ascorbate and that they also have antioxidant properties.

Dr Mark Levine of the National Institute of Health in the USA has studied the effects of vitamin C on white blood cells. His work has shown that vitamin C is critical to the disease-fighting ability of white blood cells. Research by Dr Linus Pauling supports this conclusion.

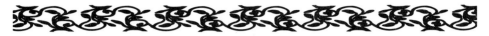

He found that the level of vitamin C in white blood cells is closely related to the body's ability to combat infection.

Vitamin C is found in citrus fruits, green vegetables, potatoes and fruit juice, so an adequate consumption of these foods will go a long way towards boosting the immune system.

Vitamin E

Vitamin E (also known as *d-alpha tocopherol*) is crucial for good health. As an enzyme-independent antioxidant, it plays a particular role in protecting the fats in cell walls. (These fats, known as *lipids*, are particularly susceptible to oxidation by free radicals.)

As an antioxidant, vitamin E has a myriad of vital functions. It stabilises membranes and protects them against free radical damage. It protects the eyes, skin, liver, breast and calf muscle tissues. Of particular importance to asthmatics is its ability to protect the lungs from oxidative damage (caused by air pollutants). It also protects and enhances the body's store of vitamin A. Vitamin E itself is enhanced by other antioxidants, such as vitamin C, and the mineral selenium.

Foods rich in vitamin E include cold-pressed oils (wheatgerm, safflower, sunflower and soyabean oils), nuts and seeds, asparagus, spinach, broccoli, butter, bananas and strawberries.

Vitamin A And Beta Carotene

The mucous membranes in our eyes, ears, nose, throat and lungs all require vitamin A to maintain their stability. Allergens can be kept at bay if the membranes are healthy.

The first fat-soluble vitamin ever to be identified, vitamin A is the general name for a group of substances which include retinol, retinal and the carotenoids. The active forms of vitamin A are found in animal tissue. The carotenoids and retinoids need bile and fats to be present in the intestines in order to be absorbed.

Although this vitamin is stable in light and heat, it is destroyed by the sun's ultraviolet rays and by oxidation, hence the need for vitamin E to be present as well, since it sacrifices itself to protect vitamin A.

Beta carotene, derived from vegetable sources, is sometimes referred to as *provitamin A*. It is found in the yellow pigment present in many fruits and vegetables. Except for diabetics, the human body can readily convert beta carotene into vitamin A. Beta carotene is

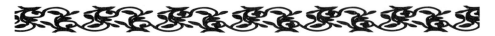

thought to be a free radical quencher, and so can protect delicate cells from the danger of oxidation.

Vitamin A is found in eggs, milk, lamb's liver, halibut liver oil, cod liver oil, dairy products, pig's kidney, beef, mackerel and canned sardines. You will find beta carotene in spinach, kale, broccoli, peaches, apricots -- the orange and green vegetables and fruits.

Zinc

Zinc is found in alpha macroglobulin, which is an important protein in the body's immune system. It follows that a shortage of the mineral will have severe consequences. What's more, zinc can actually help the immune system by clearing certain toxic metals (cadmium and lead, present in car exhaust fumes) from the body .

Its presence is also essential for normal cell division and function, and it has other cell-protecting properties apart from its antioxidant ones. In fact, zinc is involved in more enzymatic reactions than any other trace mineral.

Zinc is found in dairy products, beef, chicken, white fish and wholemeal bread. It is an all-round valuable nutrient, so make sure your intake is satisfactory. A common sign of zinc deficiency is white marks on the fingernails.

Selenium

Its name derived from the Greek moon goddess, Selene, this antioxidant trace mineral was first regarded as a poison until the discovery that it was actually needed to prevent the degeneration of liver tissue.

Vitamin B_6

Vitamin B_6 regulates antibodies and improves the activity of the T- and B-cells in the immune system. In one study, patients reported a dramatic decrease in the frequency and severity of wheezing and asthmatic attacks while taking vitamin B_6 supplements.

Vitamin B_{12}

This vitamin appears to be especially effective in sulphite-sensitive individuals. In one clinical trial, weekly injections of 1 mg of vitamin B_{12} produced a definite improvement in asthmatic patients.

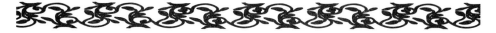

Evening Primrose Oil

The secret behind the oil of this unassuming flower lies in its gamma linolenic acid (GLA) content. Most vegetable oils contain linoleic acid, which the body has to convert into GLA. People who are atopic may be unable to convert linoleic acid into GLA. They are thought to be deficient in a particular enzyme that is needed for the conversion process. In turn, GLA is used to produce a hormone-like anti-inflammatory substance called PGE1 (prostaglandin) which stimulates the T-suppressor cells that prevent the exaggerated immune response in atopic asthma and hay fever. The high content of GLA already present in evening primrose oil can short cut the conversion process of linoleic acid into GLA and provide GLA directly to the body, thereby boosting the formation of PGE1.

Garlic

There is more to the humble bulb of this plant than just folklore. Garlic possesses antiviral properties. It can also enhance the activity of the lymphocytes thus helping the immune function which is central to all allergies. A Florida pathologist, Dr T. Abdulla, demonstrated the effect of garlic on natural killer cells. Dr Abdullah randomly divided volunteers into three groups. Over a three-week period, one group took raw garlic, one group took *aged garlic* extract and the third group took no garlic at all (the control group). At the end of the three weeks, Dr Abdullah took blood samples from each volunteer and tested the natural killer cells in the blood against tumour cells in test tubes. The natural killer cells of those who took raw garlic killed 139 per cent more tumour cells than those of the control group. And the natural killer cells of those who took aged garlic extract killed 159 per cent more tumour cells than those in the control group.

Magnesium

This trace mineral is known to improve breathing in asthmatics significantly, and is generally considered to be helpful to patients who suffer acute attacks of asthma.

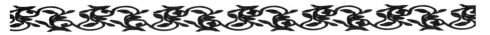

Supplements For Hay Fever And Asthma

The best source of the nutrients described is a wholefood diet. But if you are unable to obtain them from food, supplements can help to increase your intake of these nutrients up to the required levels. However, before you start taking copious amounts of antioxidant nutrients, consult a dietary therapist.

The best way to boost your nutrient intake is, generally, to take a good multivitamin mineral supplement. For more specific needs, as in hay fever or asthma, it would be well worth consulting a nutritional counsellor or a dietary therapist for a specific programme of supplements.

A Supplements Programme

- beta carotene, 15 mg per day
- vitamin B_6, 50 to 100 mg twice a day
- vitamin B_{12}, up to 500 mcg per day
- vitamin C, 1000 to 2,000 mg per day
- vitamin E, 400 iu per day
- magnesium, 400 mg per day
- selenium, 250 mcg per day
- evening primrose oil, 2 to 3 g per day
- fish oils, 1 to 2 g per day
- aged garlic extract, 1g per day.

Nutrients For The Immune System

Vitamin A And Beta Carotene
- responsible for growth and for maintaining an active thymus gland and, hence, a strong immune system
- a powerful antiviral agent – strengthens the linings in areas of special risk, for example, the gut and respiratory system.

Vitamin C
- an antiviral agent
- boosts prostaglandin E (PGE) production and increases T-lymphocyte production
- needed for collagen formation
- detoxifies many bacterial toxins
- necessary for antibody response

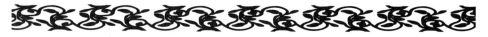

Vitamin E
- neutralises free radicals
- works with other nutrients to improve resistance to infections
- protects from air pollution

Iron
- essential for antibody production
- required for the enzyme peroxidase, which is used in the formation of white blood cells

Selenium
- a good antioxidant – it works with vitamin E
- protects against cancer-causing substances
- used in antibody production
- white cells seem to lose their ability to recognise invaders without it

Zinc
- needed for enzymes which destroy cancer cells
- thymulin, the hormone necessary for maturation of T-cells, is dependent on zinc

Antinutrients That Affect The Immune System

Fluoride
- slows the immune system
- reduces the white cells' ability to destroy foreign cells

Mercury
- adversely affects the body's ability to fight off infection
- affects the brain and the nervous system

Cadmium
- inhibits the function of some enzymes containing antibodies

Aluminium
- interferes with calcium utilisation and compromises bone function and immune function
- affects haemoglobin production

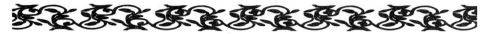

Finding A Practitioner

The British Naturopathic and Osteopathic Association, 6 Netherall Gardens, London, NW3 5 RR, maintains a register of qualified practitioners who have followed a four-year course at the British College of Naturopathy and Osteopathy.

The British Society for Nutritional Medicine, 4 Museum Street, York, YO1 2ES, maintains a register of qualified medical professionals as well as associate members who are qualified members of the related professions.

The Nutrition Association, 36 Wycombe Road, Marlow, Buckinghamshire, SL7 3HX, maintains a register of practitioners of nutrition and diet therapy.

The Nutrition Consultants Association, c/o The Institute of Optimum Nutrition, 5 Jerdan Street, London, SW6 IBE.

The Society for the Promotion of Nutritional Therapy, First Floor, The Enterprise Centre, Station Parade, Eastbourne, BN1 1BE.

Further Reading

Naturopathic Medicine by Roger Newman Turner (Thorsons).
Asthma and Bronchitis by Jan De Vries (Mainstream Publishing).
Vitamin Guide by Hasnain Walji (Element Books).
E for Additives by Maurice Hanssen (Thorsons).

4

HERBS: NATURE'S PHARMACY

Many thousands of herbs are used for medicines and among their number are those which help to relieve the symptoms of asthma and hay fever.

Herbal medicine has its origins in the time when humankind first discovered that a particular plant cured an affliction or helped to relieve pain. The Hammurabi medical code, engraved in stone around 2,000 BC, records that liquorice is useful for asthma. The Assyrian physicians were employing the same herb for 'harshness of chest'. The Egyptians and the Romans were adept at using herbs. Indeed, the builders of the Egyptian pyramids took a daily ration of garlic to ward off fevers and infections. However, the most sophisticated users of herbal medicine were the Indian and Chinese peoples, and their techniques have been passed down over the centuries and are used today. Indian Ayurvedic medicine is heavily dependent on the use of herbs and is an important form of healing.

In the Western world the use of herbs was common, too. In medieval times, all monasteries cultivated herb gardens, and since the development of the printing press in the fifteenth century, a great number of publications on herbal remedies have been produced. Herbal medicine was the chief form of medicine in the West right up until the technological and chemical advances of modern pharmacy in the nineteenth century. Thereafter, the use of synthetically manufactured drugs took the place of herbal remedies.

In 1864, a number of herbalists founded the National Association (later Institute) of Medical Herbalists. In its earlier days and to this day, this association has had to resist attempts from orthodox medical pressure groups wanting to ban herbal medicine. While it is beyond the scope of this book to discuss the issues in the modern context, the battle continues, but the Natural Medicines Society, among others, is very ably working to ensure that the right of the consumer to choose which system of medicine he or she prefers is not taken away.

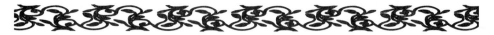

What is absurd about the controversy is that orthodox medicine has its roots in herbal medicine. Many of the synthesised drugs originate from plant materials. Steroids, for example, are synthesised from a chemical extracted from the wild yam, and the common painkiller, aspirin, was discovered in the last century in plants such as meadowsweet and willow. Today's medical profession regards plants as a source of active ingredients, which they analyse, synthesise and use in potent drugs.

However, it is the increasing use of chemically-manufactured drugs, some of which have produced unfortunate side-effects, that has led to a movement back to herbal medicine – to a rediscovery of remedies which are whole-plant based and, therefore, less prone to producing dangerous side-effects. The World Health Organisation (WHO) currently estimates that, worldwide, herbalism is three to four times more commonly practised than 'conventional' medicine.

A Holistic Approach

Just as symptoms can vary from person to person, so must herbs be chosen according to the person's disposition and symptoms. Each herb has its own therapeutic property, and medical herbalists have centuries of experience to fall back on in identifying these healing properties.

Herbal medicine differs from orthodox medicine not just because of the type of 'medicine' used, but in the general approach, that good health is not simply absence of disease but rather it is a positive state of well-being. Consequently, herbal medicine aims not merely to relieve the symptoms of disease, but also to treat the root cause of the problem itself, often by creating the conditions that mobilise the body to exercise its own capacity for healing.

Holistic herbalism is about considering the 'whole' person. Herbs are used in conjunction with a therapy that encompasses not only the physical but also the mental and spiritual aspects of treatment. Thus a holistic therapist would consider it important to have regard to the social and economic conditions that perpetuate ill health. Particular emphasis is given to fitting the treatment to the needs of the individual.

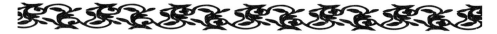

What Is A Herb?

We usually think of herbs as being plants used in cooking to add flavour, or in cosmetics, or in home remedies for their medicinal properties. To a botanist, a herb is a nonwoody plant that is under 30 cm high, while to the gardener, herbs are ornamental plants used as decoration in a herbaceous border. However, to a medical herbalist, a herb is any plant material that can be used in medicine and health care. So not only are botanical herbs used in herbal medicine, but all anatomical parts of plants including seeds, the bark of trees, flowers, ferns, mosses, fungi and seaweed.

Herbal medicines can be found in many different forms and their range of use is very wide. Homoeopathy, naturopathy,(which includes all forms of health care that cleanse and strengthen the body so as to prevent disease and maintain a state of optimum health) iridiology (a system of diagnosis whereby one can read the general body condition and the state of every organ in the body from the eye) and aromatherapy, as well as straightforward herbal medicine, all rely on herbal plants in their treatments. Western medical herbalists usually use a combination of herbs for a specific condition, although single, 'simple', herbs are also used. Other systems, especially Chinese herbalism, include prescriptions made in carefully formulated combinations. Of course, there are also the 'fast-food' herbs available in tablet form from health food shops. Herbal preparations are not only ingested orally as pills. Herbal tisanes (infusions of leaves or flowers) and teas are common, as are herbal baths. Herbal medication can be taken in the form of syrups or extraction drops to be held under the tongue where they can be absorbed quickly through the mucous tissues. Herbs can also be inhaled through steam inhalation.

How Does Herbal Medicine Work?

In common with other alternative health systems, explaining exactly how herbal medicine works is difficult. Some things work and yet there is as yet, no scientific evidence as to why they work. In general, it can be said that herbal medicines are thought to work by triggering off physiological responses which help the body to recover its normal balance, or healthy function. By taking moderate doses for long enough, these responses should become automatic, even after stopping taking the herbs.

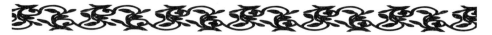

Herb formulas (as the compound medicines are known) fulfil three basic functions – as laxatives, diuretics (agents that increase the flow of urine) and blood purifiers – helping the body to eliminate and detoxify itself. They also help to keep the body in good condition by stimulating the body's own self-healing powers, thereby countering any physical symptoms, and they can build up health by toning the organs and nourishing the tissues and blood.

Herbal practitioners consider that natural remedies are safer than allopathic (orthodox) medicines because allopathic medicines are chemically synthesised and, being concentrated drugs, run the risk of producing side-effects. Herbal compounds are less likely to produce such effects as they are not only less potent, but also contain substances created naturally within the herb that may neutralise any potential dangers of the active ingredient in the plant. Herbalists do not claim that all herbal medicines are entirely free from side-effects, as many are known to be toxic if taken in high doses, but they are generally considered to be far safer than orthodox (allopathic) medicines.

Herbs And The Respiratory System

Herbal medicine is able to relieve and alleviate many aspects of disorders of the respiratory system, including asthma and hay fever.

Better breathing is achieved by strengthening the mucous membranes to ensure that vital gas exchange through these membranes can occur. Herbs can stimulate the secretions in the lung tissue so that the air is sufficiently moistened and the membranes are protected. Herbs also work to tone up the circulation by ensuring that blood bathes the tissues properly and, by stimulating the whole of the glandular and excretory processes, they help to produce a clean and harmonious inner environment which facilitates a sound respiratory system. This all means that herbs can act either as respiratory stimulants or respiratory relaxants, according to the need of the patient.

Herbs also act as demulcents, which means that they can allay irritation, and as amphoteric remedies, which means that how they work depends on the circumstances, changing and adapting if necessary. In other words, they act as normalisers.

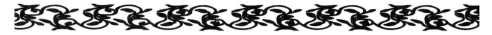

Asthma

Many possible causes of asthma are considered when a herbal medicine is to be prescribed. There is usually an allergic component, which triggers an asthmatic attack, while the problem may also be genetic or the result of continued exposure to an irritant. Other factors to be considered include diet, lifestyle and the associated pressures of tension, anxiety and exhaustion. It is, therefore, difficult to describe one or even a few herbal compounds which deal exclusively with asthma.

Herbalists generally look at particular symptoms and suggest remedies. For example, herbs that are known to help reduce spasm are Grindelia, Lobelia, Mouse Ear, Pill Bearing Spurge, Sundew, Wild Cherry Bark and Elecampane. Catarrhal build-up may be treated with White Horehound, Blood Root and Coltsfoot. To get rid of sputum, expectorants, such as Aniseed, Coltsfoot or Liquorice, are effective, while heart strength can be boosted through the use of the herb Motherwort. Anxiety and tension, so common in asthmatics, can be treated with Hops, Skullcap or Valerian. Garlic, too, is widely recognised as having universal usage as an antimicrobial preventive for respiratory infections, and is thought of as a substance that will augment the body's health as well as being a general protector.

Hay Fever

Medicinal herbs for the alleviation of hay fever and its symptoms include Coneflower, which promotes natural immunity, increases general resistance and acts as a blood purifier. Garlic is a natural antiseptic and blood purifier. Breathing problems and catarrh are eased with the use of Coltsfoot, which is soothing and helps to remove obstructive phlegm, as does Mullein. Elderflower promotes sweating and urination, essential for the cleansing process, and is useful for a hay fever case with a background of sinus congestion. Golden Rod stimulates the mucous membranes and is particularly effective in cases of catarrh with sneezing and mucus build-up. Hyssop is an invaluable cough medicine and soothes inflamed membranes (it should not be taken in pregnancy). Yarrow is also a tonic for the membranes and is useful for feverish conditions. Other hay fever symptoms, such as an irritable throat or nose and sore eyes, can be treated with the herb Eyebright, and Red Sage may be

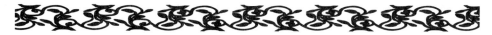

used as a mouth lotion or gargle for pharyngitis and a sore throat. Combinations of herbs in the form of compounds which are to be infused can work on various aspects of hay fever.

For acute hay fever with a runny nose and itchy eyes, a combination of Coneflower, Euphrasia and Golden Rod is useful, while a combination of Elderflower, Mullein, Hyssop, Yarrow and Coltsfoot can help a tight chest, wheezy cough and mucus build-up. A long-term treatment programme for starting in early spring and continuing throughout the hay fever season is made up of a combination of Coneflower and Mullein to help build general resistance and to tone the mucous membranes. Coneflower, Elderflower, Mullein and Yarrow taken together, will aid general detoxification and cleansing.

The Medical Herbalist

A medical herbalist can give more specialist advice on the use of herbal medicines. He or she is trained to carry out a full medical examination, similar to that which a doctor would give. After the diagnosis, the herbalist prescribes what combination of herbs is needed and whether it should be taken in the form of a tincture (a medicinal extract in a solution of alcohol), liquid supplement or infusion.

The herbalist will normally ask you about your lifestyle and diet in some detail. He or she will also explain to you that treatment is aimed at helping the body to enhance its own healing potential. Elimination of toxins is a fundamental part of the treatment, and the remedies work slowly. He or she will probably advise you to be patient if you are one of those people who expect to feel better 10 minutes after taking a pill.

Some Commonly Used Herbs And Combinations For Asthma And Hay Fever

Angelica *(Angelica sinesis) Chinese angelica.* Particularly suitable for those who are sensitive to pollens, dust, animal dander and other airborne particles. In fact, this herb has had a long history of use by Chinese herbalists in the management of allergies because of its ability to inhibit the production of antibodies.

Chinese Skullcap *(Scutellaria baicalensis).* This herb is used for its anti-inflammatory properties. It has a high flavonoid content. This inhibits the formation of certain other compounds in the body which

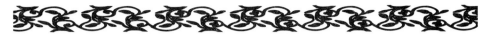

have an even worse effect than histamine. Flavonoids also act as antioxidants and as powerful free radical scavengers.

Coltsfoot (Tussilago farfara). Tussilago means 'cough dispeller'. This is a powerful expectorant that also has soothing qualities. It has proved to be especially useful for the elderly as it helps to bring up mucus and relieve a tight chest. Chinese herbalists recommend a tea made of Coltsfoot leaves (Chinese name: K'uan-tung) with Fenugreek seeds and crushed fresh Ginger Root for the relief of wheezing, stubborn coughs and irritations of the lungs and air passages.

Chamomile (Anthemis nobilis). A very popular herb for many complaints, this is a useful remedy to be given in an asthma attack because of its antispasmodic, as well as sedative, properties. It can be taken frequently for breathing difficulties and is considered particularly useful for babies and young children.

Ephedra (Ephedra sinica). In the Chinese herbal tradition, the medicinal use of this herb can be traced back to 5,000 years ago. The Chinese have long favoured Ephedra for allergy and inflammatory conditions. Modern medicine 'discovered' the alkaloid compound, ephedrine, in 1923, and soon began to manufacture it synthetically. It is used together with related compounds in many prescription medicines for asthma and hay fever. Prolonged use of the herb is thought to weaken the adrenal glands and so it is necessary to combine it with other herbs and nutrients that support the adrenal glands, such as Liquorice, Panax Ginseng, vitamin C, magnesium, zinc and vitamin B_6. The traditional herbal combinations of asthma and hay fever remedies involve the use of Ephedra with expectorants, such as Lobelia, Grindelia and Euphorbia. This herb is only available when prescribed by a medical herbalist.

Euphorbia (Euphorbia hirta). Also known as the asthma weed, this herb relieves spasm. It is considered particularly useful for the chronic asthmatic as it can prevent an asthma spasm from occurring if a regular dose is taken before a meal.

Ginko (Ginko biloba). The name 'Ginko' is a Chinese word meaning 'silver fruit' which is highly prized in China. The tree has a peculiar and a mysterious immunity to diseases which attack other trees, and is classified as one of the oldest living species of tree. Popularly known for its medicinal properties that can quickly cure the common cold, it has also been found to be effective in relieving nasal congestion, stubborn coughs and asthma. For asthmatics, Chinese herbalists recommend a formula containing Ginko seeds (known as Pai-kuo) and nine assistant herbs.

Liquorice (Glycyrrhiza glabra) (Chinese name Kan-ts'ao). Well known for its anti-inflammatory and anti-allergy properties, it is a popular medicine for chest and lung complaints. It is also used as a base for mixing herbs.

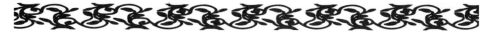

Chinese herbalists consider it to be a harmonising ingredient in a large number of prescriptions. Its activity in asthma and hay fever is due to its ability to increase the anti-inflammatory action of the hormone cortisol. Liquorice has a similar action to cortisone, a widely-used drug in the treatment of asthma, in reducing inflammation through its ability to inhibit the activity of several enzymes involved. Liquorice is also thought to help reduce some of the significant side-effects associated with cortisone.

Lobelia *(Lobelia inflata)*. Also known as Indian Tobacco, this herb is found in a number of asthma formulas. It is both an expectorant and an antispasmodic, and has been found to work very quickly. It helps to relax the bronchial muscle by promoting the release of adrenal hormones. Lobelia is only available over the counter in tablet (compound) form.

Finding A Practitioner

Professional Medical Herbalists

Practitioners are usually members of the National Institute of Medical Herbalists and apply Western herbal medicine in a consulting room. The diagnostic techniques of many qualified medical herbalists resemble those of GPs, using the same methods and equipment for blood pressure, pulse taking, physical examination and assessment of urine and blood samples.
The National Institute of Medical Herbalists, 9, Palace Gate, Exeter EX1 1JA.
The General Council and Register of Consultant Herbalists, Marlborough House, Swanpool, Falmouth, Cornwall, TR11 4HW.

Chinese Herbalists

Traditional Chinese herbalists practise mainly within the Chinese community. 'Modern' practitioners of Chinese herbalism often use herbs in conjunction with acupuncture.
Register of Chinese Herbal Medicine, 138 Prestbury Road, Cheltenham GLS2 2DP.

Ayrvedic and Unani Practitioners

Commonly known as *Vaids* and *Hakims*, these practitioners are mainly found within the Indian and Pakistani communities and offer treatment on traditional principles.

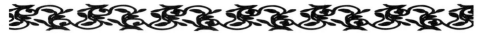

Further Reading

A-Z of Modern Herbalism by Simon Mills (Thorsons).
Herbalism: Headway Lifeguides by Frances Büning and Paul
   Hambly (Hodder & Stoughton).
Herbal Medicine by Dian Dincin Buchman (Rider Books).
Potter's New Cyclopaedia of Botanical Drogs, by R C Wren (C W Daniel).
Thorson's Guide to Medical Herbalism by David Hoffman (Thorsons).
The New Holistic Herbal by David Hoffman (Element Books).
Traditional Home Herbal Remedies by Jan de Vries (Mainstream
   Publishing).

HOMOEOPATHY: LIKE CURES LIKE

Paracelsus, a sixteenth-century philosopher and physician, said, 'Those who merely study and treat the effects of disease are like those who imagine that they can drive away winter by brushing snow from the door. It is not the snow that causes winter, but winter that causes the snow.' Good homoeopathy will not just drive away the symptoms of disease but will help patients deal with the cause of illness and regain their health. A homoeopath's ultimate aim is for the patient to reach a level of health free from dependency on any medicine or therapy.

In common with many other natural therapies, homoeopathy regards illness as a sign of imbalance, and treatment seeks to address the underlying reasons for an ailment rather than merely to deal with the symptoms. From the homoeopathic point of view, allergic conditions, such as hay fever and asthma, are seen as reflecting an imbalance in the immune system itself. Treatment is, therefore, aimed at restoring balance and freeing the immune system from its oversensitive state.

Homoeopathic preparations are actually highly diluted forms of substances which, in a full-strength dose, would produce symptoms of a disease in a healthy person. For example, *Arsenicum,* a proven remedy for hay fever sufferers, is a preparation of a minute quantity of arsenic trioxide – a poison that induces severe burning and prickly symptoms in the membranes. The more closely a preparation imitates a person's symptoms, the more effective it is.

Homoeopathy is a system of medicine based on the natural law *Similia similibus curentur* ('Like cures like'). This principle was known to Hippocrates and Paracelsus, but credit is usually given to Samuel Hahnemann, a German doctor of the late eighteenth century. He believed that human beings have an innate capacity to heal themselves, and that the symptoms of disease reflect the individual's struggle to overcome the forces antagonistic to life. The physician's work must be to discover and, if possible, remove the cause of the trouble, and to stimulate the vital healing force of nature.

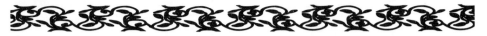

Inspired by the discovery that a herbal remedy for malaria, chinchona tree bark, actually produced symptoms of the disease, such as headache and intermittent fever, Hahnemann and his followers carried out experiments on themselves called 'provings' in which, over long periods, they took small doses of various poisonous or medicinal substances and carefully noted the symptoms they produced. Patients suffering from similar symptoms were then treated with these substances with very encouraging results.

Hahnemann worked to establish the smallest possible dose and he increasingly diluted the medicine, for he realised that this was the best way to avoid side-effects. By accident, he found that, using a special method of succussion (vigorous shaking), combined with dilution, it became more effective, provided it matched the symptoms of the patient.

How Homoeopathy Works

Homoeopaths regard symptoms as an adaptive response by the body in defending itself and as a sign of disease. Allopathic (orthodox) practitioners, on the other hand, see the symptoms as the disease. A homoeopath looks at the symptoms as the way in which the body expresses its reaction to the underlying disorder. His or her task is to prescribe a remedy that will stimulate the body to heal itself more quickly. The yardstick of a correct remedy is one that will create similar symptoms in a healthy person when given in material dosages. A very apt description was given by the German national homoeopathic organisation: 'The determination as to whether or not a remedy is homoeopathic is derived neither from its amount nor from its form, but solely from its relation to the disease' (the law of similars).

The homoeopathic doctrine rests on three principles:

The Law of Similars

Homoeopaths regard all symptoms of a patient's condition – mental, emotional and physical – as evidence of a unified effort to resolve an inner disturbance and to return to a state of balance. The homoeopath selects and prescribes a remedy which, through previous testing on healthy people and from clinical experience, is known to produce a similar symptom picture to that of the patient. The prescribed similar remedy then stimulates and assists the patient's own natural healing efforts.

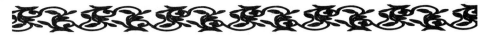

The Single Remedy

Symptoms often appear to be localised, but it is the patient's whole system which is out of balance and is striving to return to health. This whole can only be stimulated by a single remedy at any one time. The prescription of a single remedy allows the homoeopath to evaluate its effect.

The Minimal Dose

Because of the similarity of the remedy's known 'symptom picture' to that of the patient's, the patient is highly sensitive to its stimulus, and so only a minute dose is needed in the form of a specially prepared potency. The potency and number of doses is determined by the homoeopath according to the needs of the individual patient.

It is the concept of dilution that has caused the debate as to whether homoeopathy is a valid therapy. Homoeopathic remedies are diluted to such a degree that hardly any of the original substance is left at all. How can such a remedy work?

Most homoeopaths readily admit that they do not know, but are quick to point out that the remedy works and are content to leave it at that. Some say that to look for a physical explanation is to miss the point. It could well be that these high potencies may be acting at a subtle level of energy, like the *chi* in Chinese medicine or the *prana* in Ayurvedic medicine – the 'vital force'. A healthy person vibrates at a certain energy frequency which is more harmonious than that of an unhealthy person. The right homoeopathic remedy is like a boost of subtle energy which returns the body to its proper energy frequency. A body that is in tune – resonating at its proper rate – is able to use its immune system to throw off the toxins that cause illness.

How Homoeopathic Remedies Are Made

When we cut a strong onion we often experience an acrid, runny nose, soreness in the throat and stinging, runny eyes. A homoeopath may prescribe a remedy called *Allium cepa* (made from onion) for the patient who has a cold with these particular symptoms. Homoeopathic medicines can be prepared from anything which causes symptoms, and so they come from many sources. Most are derived from plants, but minerals, metals and some animals are also used.

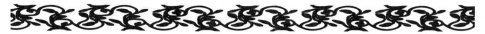

After the raw materials have been prepared, the remedies are made by a number of dilutions and succussion. Each stage of succussion increases the potency, which is given a number and a letter. Potencies with an 'X' affix are diluted 1:9 at each successive stage, and those with a 'C' affix are diluted similarly, but in the ratio of 1:99.

The more a remedy is diluted, the stronger it becomes, that is, the more energy it possesses, and the more capable it is of dealing with the root cause of the problem. It is common for homoeopaths to use strengths such as 200C and 10M ('M' being used to denote 1000C). These high doses are usually used to treat chronic disease, and are said to act on a subtle energy level as well as the physical body.

Homoeopathic remedies should be protected from contamination. They should not be touched, exposed to sunlight, stored near strong-smelling substances or taken near meals or drinks as their energy can easily be negated.

How The Remedies Are Given

Most health food stores and chemists only stock low potencies, such as the sixth (a six times dilution), for example, Arnica 6. High-potency remedies are usually only prescribed by experienced and qualified homoeopaths.

Remedies can be administered in different ways. Sometimes they are given in a single dose in high potency form. Or the homoeopath may decide to give a remedy with a low potency, but repeated frequently.

> The homoeopath will choose the method to suit the patient and the nature of the illness. For instance, a person who has been ill for a long time and whose body has been physically damaged may need repeated doses of a remedy to stimulate the recuperative powers, whereas a young, basically healthy, person may respond very quickly to a single, high-potency remedy. Individual patients also respond better to some methods than others; understanding this is part of the skill of the homoeopath and explains why attempts to self-prescribe may prove ineffective.
>
> *(The Society of Homoeopaths)*

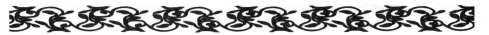

Consulting A Homoeopathic Practitioner

Experienced homoeopaths have undergone at least three years of study. At the first consultation, the practitioner will take a detailed personal history. You will be asked many questions about your past and present medical history and what type of person you are – whether you prefer a hot or a cold climate, whether you are a sympathetic person, and about your likes and dislikes, for example. He or she will look at your appearance and manner, and try to assess your physical and mental states. Your personal circumstances, anxieties, fears and beliefs and self-confidence are all important aspects in the diagnosis. Usually, he or she will send you home with a single dose prescription and ask you to come back after four to six weeks.

During treatment – as with other natural therapies – you may experience a slight 'spring cleaning' of the body, perhaps in the form of a cold. The body is getting rid of the toxins naturally, and this process should not be interfered with unless absolutely necessary. Also, someone with a long history of different illnesses may re-experience these slightly in the reverse order in which they occurred.

A Conversation With A Homoeopathic Practitioner

Q. What are the goals of homoeopathic treatment?
A. The goal is to get you to a level of health, of balance and freedom from limitations so that you eventually need only very infrequent medication.

Q. Why do homoeopaths ask so many questions?
A. Constitutional homoeopathy does not treat specific diseases as such, but treats individuals. Hence a detailed understanding of the patient is fundamental to making a correct prescription.
The homoeopath must attempt an almost impossible task – that of coming quickly to a complete understanding of an individual. The questioning process is essential for forming and developing this understanding.
The homoeopath needs to be an acute listener and observer – our job is primarily to get your symptom picture and match this to a remedy. So we

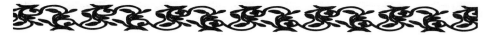

want to hear your story and listen sympathetically, without making any value judgements, and match this information to the right remedy.

To match a remedy to an individual, we must know all the person's limitations clearly: this includes mental, emotional and physical levels, and such aspects as general energy, effects of the environment, and causative factors.

Q. How many appointments are necessary?
A. In the beginning (that is, in the first six months) visits may be more frequent and will taper off as you become healthier. We feel we need to see you initially more frequently (follow-ups are usually every four to six weeks in the beginning) to work with you and evaluate your progress. Yet we are not insensitive to the cost of treatment, and do not wish to make this a burden.

If a remedy has acted curatively, even in deep and complex cases, after the initial follow-up we may not need to see you for some time. This is because the remedy has brought your system into balance and, in our experience, this state can last for a long time. We also need to wait until the next 'remedy picture' comes up clearly. This is the time to have a renewed faith in your body's healing abilities.

Q. How can I be involved?
A. You don't have to believe in homoeopathic remedies in order for them to work (we treat babies and there are homoeopathic vets). But to select the correct remedy and for the treatment to continue to act, your co-operation and commitment is necessary.

You can help by:

- Noting any changes after you take the remedy – keeping a weekly journal can be helpful for bringing to your follow-up consultations. Please note general changes as well as specific ones.
- Being clear and complete about your symptoms on all levels.
- A commitment to a long-term process and perspective is really a commitment to your long-term well-being.
- Above all, communicating any concerns or questions you may have. We are always trying to find better ways of helping you and welcome your comments.

Q. How do homoeopaths evaluate a curative response?
A. Homoeopaths have, through over 170 years of experience, developed sophisticated means of evaluating curative responses, and have established laws and principles of cure.

On a simpler level, you want to see the problems you have come with clear up, and they should. Always keep in mind that ours is a total perspective on you, and we want to see overall improvements as well as

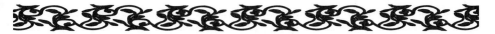

specific ones. You also have to see improvement in the context of the amount of stress in your life. So improvements will occur on physical, emotional and mental levels, and in general energy. Observe and report these general changes as well as specific ones.

Q. How long does treatment take?

A. This is a difficult question to answer, but after several interviews the homoeopath is better able to give you an idea of this. In simpler problems and in acute situations, results can begin quickly and dramatically.

For a small percentage of relatively healthy individuals, one or two treatments may be all that is needed to stabilise the system for years at a stretch, but such an ideal would, for most people, be an unrealistic expectation.

Q. Should I come back after I am feeling better?

A. The four-to-six week follow-up is important to return for. After you are feeling consistently better, we would like to see you for regular check-ups to prevent future problems. Usually, this is at four-to-six month intervals.

Q. Where are the remedies from?

A. We either have your remedy available at the clinic and will dispense it, the cost usually being included in your consultation fee, or we shall refer you to a convenient homoeopathic supplier.

For more information about specific remedies, their origin and nature, refer to the reading list at the end of this chapter.

Q. How can a few doses do anything or last a long time?

A. The remedies are highly potent – they are prepared in what is called a 'potentised dilution' and dropped on to tiny lactose granules, pillules, tablets or powders. They simply catalyse or trigger a response by the body on an energetic level, rather than effect chemical change. So, ultimately, what works better after the remedy is taken is your own regulating system. The remedy helps the body develop a natural, positive momentum which continues to gain strength and eliminate disease.

Should you want to gain a more in-depth understanding of this fascinating and profound process, refer to any of the books on the reading list.

Q. Is there any advice about diet and lifestyle?

A. The homoeopath doesn't always give advice about lifestyle and diet. A good diet is, of course, essential for a healthy body. Any advice about diet and exercise is tailored to the individual's own needs in terms of their illness, age and various environmental factors. This is because we always want to see clearly whether the homoeopathic remedy alone is working.

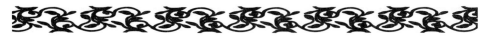

Also, we believe that when the organism is healthy an imbalanced lifestyle will diminish and positive changes will permeate all aspects of your life. There may be obvious 'obstacles to cure' in your life or environment which the homoeopath will discuss with you.

Q. Can homoeopathy work in more complex or chronic cases, and how long does it take?

A. In more complex cases, homoeopathic treatment is like peeling away the layers of an onion. Briefly, this means that we build up layers of symptoms, or 'pathology', as a response to certain stresses as we go through life. These layers are laid down and can be peeled away effectively with homoeopathic remedies. During treatment, old sets of symptoms may come up (but because with each successive remedy you are healthier, they will not be as severe as in the past). A recurrence of an old set of symptoms may be the indication for a new remedy to be given. Even some hereditary tendencies can be eliminated with homoeopathy.

So in deep or chronic problems the curative process may be gradual, and consultations more frequent.

Q. What happens if the symptoms seem to return?

A. If you had a good curative response to a remedy and then after, say, two to six months (or at any time) a relapse seems to occur, we usually recommend waiting a few days to see if your system re-balances itself. If any severe symptoms develop, do not wait. If the symptoms persist after a week, then a repeat of the remedy may be necessary. If so, another appointment would be needed.

Do not get disappointed or discouraged at this point and feel that homoeopathy is not working for you – this is just a phase of getting you to a consistently good state of health.

This situation may mean a new remedy is indicated as a 'layer' of symptoms from the past comes up and needs to be treated.

Q. What will interfere with the remedy working?

A. Camphor products and highly aromatic essential oils, such as peppermint and menthol can all interfere. There are certain therapies that can interfere, such as chemical therapies (natural or otherwise), high-potency vitamins, intensive exercise programmes, and certain dental procedures. It is not usually a good idea to have acupuncture during a course of homoeopathic treatment as it interferes with the 'vital force' and both treatments are based on the premise that they work by stimulating the body's healing powers.

We have found that massage, mild chiropractic and osteopathic treatments, and certain gentle therapies or medications do not interfere

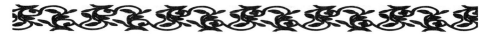

with homoeopathic treatment.

If you are considering any other therapy, consult your homoeopath first. It is also best to avoid, or at least greatly reduce, the intake of coffee and other caffeine drinks as these are said to interfere with the subtle movement of the healing force.

Q. Can a wrong remedy be given and what are the effects?
A. As carefully as we try to match the correct remedy, we do not always achieve 100 per cent accuracy. If appropriately used, homoeopathic treatment should produce no side-effects from the remedies. Either nothing changes or the true symptom picture will become even clearer and the right remedy is more obvious.

It can take several interviews for a homoeopath to get an accurate picture of the totality of your symptoms and an 'essential' understanding of this to select the right remedy. Of course, the clearer and more in touch you are with yourself, the easier this task becomes.

Q. What about seeing a GP?
A. Homoeopathy is complementary to the health care that is available. We recommend that you should maintain your relationship with your doctor, especially for routine needs and emergencies. Your GP will also arrange for you to have any blood tests or X-rays, etc. or refer you to a consultant.

Q. What about acute problems?
A. Homoeopathic remedies can be used to treat acute problems, such as flu and stomach upsets, and even help the body to heal itself after injuries and falls. If you are already having homoeopathic treatment, mild illnesses will often clear up on their own, but if the symptoms are getting worse, please phone for advice. If your symptoms are severe, phone immediately. If necessary contact your GP.

If you are involved in an accident or emergency, you should go to your nearest casualty department for treatment and then phone to see if a homoeopathic remedy is also indicated.

Hay Fever Remedies

For recurrent symptoms it is recommended that you contact a practitioner. However, you can use the following homoeopathic medicines at home during an attack.

Sabadilla. For typical symptoms of hay fever, such as watery nasal discharge, sneezing, runny eyes and itchy nose.

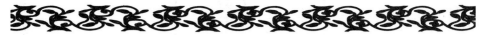

Wyethia. For itching on the back part of the roof of the mouth or itching behind the nose. Also for dryness of the nasal passages and the throat (despite a continuous watery discharge from the nose).

Allium cepa. For burning nasal discharge and profusely watering eyes which are red with burning tears.

Euphrasia. For copious burning tears and watery nasal discharge. Also for a loose cough when large amounts of mucus formed in the upper airways are coughed up.

Arsenicum. For irritation and tickling in the nose and frequent and violent sneezing that does not relieve irritation.

Asthma Remedies

For mild to moderate attacks, the following remedies may help during an attack. For long-term management of asthma, it is recommended that you consult a practitioner.

Arsenicum. The indications for the use of this remedy are fearfulness, when you cannot seem to get your breath and you are in an agitated, restless state, particularly when the symptoms of shortness of breath and wheezing worsen at night. This remedy is particularly suitable for people who are restless and anxious by nature.

Pulsatilla. For wheezing that gets worse in the evening or at night. Also for accumulation of phlegm in the chest that needs to be coughed up or for asthma that gets worse after eating rich or fatty foods. This remedy is ideally suited to people who are affectionate and often tearful by nature.

Ipecac. For wheezing and a rattling of mucus when breathing. Also for those whose asthma is accompanied by a great deal of phlegm in the chest.

Spongia. For those with dry asthma with little or no phlegm in the chest.
Breathing is noisy and shortness of breath is made worse by lying down.

Chamomilla. For those asthmatics, especially children, who display irritability and are disagreeable.

Important. You must get medical care immediately for any severe shortness of breath or sore throat with difficulty in swallowing.

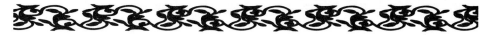

Finding A Practitioner

An increasing number of qualified medical doctors now offer homoeopathic treatment. Most of them have taken a postgraduate training course to become a Member or a Fellow of the Faculty of Homoeopathy (MSHom or FFHom). A register of these is maintained by the Faculty of Homoeopathy, c/o Royal London Homoeopathic Hospital, Great Ormond Street, London WC1N 3HR. Many of the professional homoeopaths have trained for four years at accredited colleges and have become graduate or registered members of the Society of Homoeopaths (RSHom). For a list of registered homoeopaths, write to The Society of Homoeopaths, 2 Artizan Road, Northampton NN1 4HU.

In addition to the private and NHS practitioners, there are five NHS homoeopathic hospitals in London, Bristol, Tunbridge Wells, Liverpool and Glasgow. There are also a number of private clinics nationally. Further information may be obtained from The British Homoeopathic Association, 27A Devonshire Street, London W1N 1RJ.

Further Reading

There are some excellent books available on homoeopathy. We have listed the more introductory books:

Homoeopathy: Headway Lifeguides by Beth MacEoin (Hodder & Stoughton).
Homoeopathy for Emergencies by Phyllis Speight (C W Daniels).
The Complete Homoeopathy Handbook: A Guide to Everyday Health Care by Miranda Castro (Macmillan).
The Family Guide to Homoeopathy: The Safe Form of Medicine for the Future by Andrew Lockie (Elm Tree Books).
Homoeopathy, Medicine for the New Man by George Vithoulkas (Thorsons).
Everybody's Guide to Homoeopathic Medicines by Stephen Cummings and Dana Ullman (Gollancz).
Homoeopathy: Medicine for the 21st Century by Dana Ullman (Thorsons).

6

ANTHROPOSOPHICAL MEDICINE: AN EXTENSION TO CONVENTIONAL PRACTICE

The allopathic medical approach is based on a mechanistic view of the human being. In other words, it looks at the body rather than at the person. The growth of interest in other systems of medicine bears testimony to the fact that something is lacking.

Most of the alternative and complementary approaches to healing discussed in this book are based on ancient philosophies and the value systems of the civilisations that they represent. Anthroposophical practitioners, however, believe that turning to these in search of what is lacking in conventional medicine is like trying to turn the clock back. What is needed is not a return to the past, but an extension of conventional medicine to take account of both the spiritual and the physical sides of the person.

Anthroposophical medicine offers a spiritual dimension to allopathy. Its founder, the Austrian philosopher and scientist, Rudolph Steiner (1861–1925), sought to go beyond the limits of materialism in search of the spiritual side of human existence. He believed that we are made up of body, soul and spirit and anthroposophical medicine recognises that healing must take place on all levels. The foundations of anthroposophical medicine were laid when a Dutch doctor, Ita Wegmen, in collaboration with Steiner, who was not a medical doctor himself, wrote a book called *The Fundamentals of Therapy* aimed at the medical profession. Anthroposophical medicine was to be regarded as an extension to conventional practice rather than as an alternative.

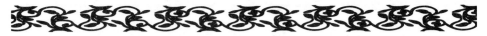

The Four Aspects Of A Complete Person

To the physical body must be added three other elements in order to complete the picture of a human being. In anthroposophical parlance, they are called the *etheric body, astral body* and *ego*. These nonmaterial elements are common to us all, but they cannot be perceived with the physical senses. Sometimes the terms *life element, soul element* and *spirit*, respectively, are used. All these three nonphysical aspects maybe described as 'spiritual', but the spirit itself is the unique inner identity.

The Anthroposophical Elements Of A Complete Person			
Spirit	Self-consciousness	Human	Ego
Soul	Consciousness	Animal	Astral body
Life	Life	Plant	Etheric body
Material	Weighable and measurable	Mineral	Physical body

The Etheric Body

The etheric body, or the life element, can best be described as that force which governs the existence of the physical body. The best illustration of how the life element works is that after death the physical body, left under the influence of physical laws, begins to deteriorate from being a highly-organised structure into dust.

Not only is the etheric body responsible for building and organising growth, it is also responsible for maintaining and repairing parts of the physical body. It is this force that strives to keep us in good health and helps the physical body to recover from less serious ailments. The etheric body's continuous fight against death and decay in the physical body must be understood in order to comprehend fully any organism and its diseases.

The Astral Body

This soul element is what differentiates humans and animals from the plant kingdom. Both humans and animals are conscious of the physical world and have instinct. We all experience pain when the physical body is hurt, but we are also aware of inner pain when someone hurts our feelings. The main difference between anthroposophical doctors and conventional doctors is that the

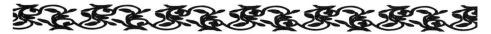

former consider the soul element as much as the physical element, while the latter rely principally on the physical.

The astral body has a *catabolic* (breaking down) effect on the physical body and, as such, has an opposite effect to the etheric body, which constantly strives to build and repair (*anabolic* effect). Anthroposophical practitioners believe that health prevails as long as the destructive process, brought about by the astral body, is held in check by the building force of the etheric body. Any imbalance between these two forces will result in disease.

Ego

Awareness of the physical world and the experience of pleasure and pain are common characteristics of animals and human beings, because they both have astral bodies. Human beings have one additional level of consciousness that animals lack. It is the ability to think, together with an awareness that they are independent, conscious beings. Anthroposophical medicine describes this as the spirit, or the ego. This dimension has a dual effect on the physical body. It works with the etheric body in its anabolic activity, and with the astral body in its catabolic activity.

The Anthroposophical View Of Illness

Anthroposophical medicine looks at illness in terms of the interrelationships between the ego, the astral body, the etheric body and the physical body. It seeks to influence the activity of one or more of these elements so as to restore balance and, therefore, health.

The three main systems within anthroposophical medicine are the nerve–sense system, the metabolic limb system and the rhythmic system.

Associated with consciousness, the *nerve–sense system* incorporates the nerves, the brain, the spinal cord and the sense organs.

The *metabolic limb system* includes the stomach, intestines and the lymphatic system. This system is characterised by unconsciousness; we are not aware of its anabolic processes unless there is something wrong and we feel pain.

In the middle of these two is the *rhythmic system,* which is centred on the heart and the lungs. The rhythmic system plays a major role in the maintenance of health as it is involved in keeping the nerve–sense and the metabolic limb systems in a state of balance.

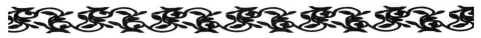

An excess in the activity of the metabolic limb system means an increase in warmth and an excess of fluid. Too much nerve–sense activity is characterised by a loss of fluid, excessive hardening, etc, which are all features of degenerative diseases. In fact, the anthroposophical system of medicine is based on two main types of illness: inflammatory or feverish on the one hand, and degenerative and hardening on the other. It follows that when illness comes about as a result of an imbalance between the nerve–sense system and the metabolic limb system, a cure can only be effected when the balance is restored. The practitioner uses different methods to achieve this.

The Three Systems In Anthroposophical Medicine			
Nerve–Sense:	Thinking	Conscious	Cooling Catabolic Hardening
Rhythmic:	Feeling	Dream-like	Balancing Mediating
Metabolic Limb:	Volition	Unconscious	Warming Anabolic Softening

Use Of Medicines

The anthroposophical doctor looks for examples in nature and bases his or her remedies on natural life processes which are similar to those in the human organism. In contrast with conventional medicine, which analyses disease in terms of molecular change and develops medicine to counteract those changes so as to alleviate the symptoms, anthroposophical medicine looks at the interplay of the processes that cause the molecular changes associated with the symptoms.

Artistic Therapies

Based on the premise that artistic activities have an impact on the consciousness of an individual, as well as society as a whole, anthroposophical practitioners have devised a number of techniques that help in healing, such as music, painting, sculpture and architecture. Music, for example, which has a powerful impact

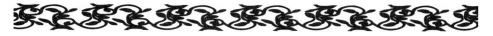

on feelings, is an expression of the laws of the spirit within the realm of the soul. In other words, the ego is expressed at the astral level. Similarly, painting is an expression of the astral in the etheric realm, and sculpture a manifestation of the etheric level in the physical body. Rudolph Steiner devised an art of movement called *eurhythmy* to express the forms of movement of the physical body in the physical realm.

Painting therapy is used to treat a number of disorders of the rhythmic system, such as asthma, in which the rhythm of breathing is impaired because the airways have been partially blocked. An anthroposophical practitioner would view this as the result of an imbalance between the airy and the watery elements, which correspond to the astral and etheric bodies respectively, and would seek to redress the predominance of the etheric (watery) activity.

Hydrotherapy And Massage

Anthroposophical practitioners may recommend hydrotherapy because water is the one medium that we all experienced before birth. It is considered to play a special role in the healing process. Indeed, the healing properties of baths have been recognised since the time of ancient Greece. It is said that Hippocrates established a healing centre which had elaborate bathing facilities on the island of Cos. Every culture has had spas and bathing centres. In Europe, the healing effects of certain springs have led to the development of spa towns, some of which still flourish today.

Rhythmic massage is another manifestation of anthroposophic practice, which seeks to balance the etheric forces with the tension created by the astral influence.

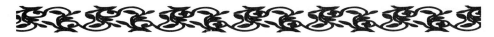

A Conversation With An Anthroposophical Doctor

Q. Where do you place asthma and hay fever in the anthroposophical system of medicine?
A. Asthma is a problem that expresses itself in the rhythmic system as it is to do with breathing and the action of the heart. Breathing incorporates two stages: breathing in and breathing out, or in-breath and out-breath. Asthma, in particular, is a difficulty in breathing out. The general direction of the therapy is, therefore, in helping the patient to breathe out. Out-breathing is the dominant gesture. Massage and application of special oils, accompanied by movement therapy are all part of the treatment.

Q. It is said that the rhythmic system is a balancing system in the body. Could you explain this ?
A. The head/nerve sense system is one sided. It is considered unhealthy because, while it is full of consciousness there is hardly any life force in it. Its biochemistry is very fickle and hovers on the brink of life. If you deprive the system of oxygen, it can die in a very short time.

On the other hand, the metabolic limb system has very little consciousness, but a wealth of life. It is not as vulnerable and there is an abundance of regeneration. For example, there is exuberance of life in our sexual organs which produce millions of cells when we just need one cell to procreate.

The rhythmic system is responsible for the balancing act between consciousness and the regenerative forces of the body required by the body for optimum health. A disorder that expresses itself in this system is therefore considered health giving.

Q. What about the immune system and allergies?
A. This really is a question of boundaries. The penetration by foreign organisms in the hay fever sufferer is the weakness of the boundaries, which are our first line of defence, because the physical level of the boundaries is not sufficiently established. Asthma is a boundary problem in the bronchi and in the allergic asthmatic the boundary simply does not exist. The integrity of the boundary is guarded by the immune system. Inflammation in hay fever is considered relatively harmless because this is a healthy and exuberant reaction by the body and a good sign of a potentially healthy immune system, just as fevers are considered a healthy response to infections. If the reaction was unnoticed and the

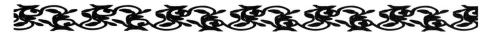

immune system was malfunctioning, for example in cancer, then it would be considered unhealthy.

Q. I understand that painting therapy is considered to be particularly therapeutic for asthma patients by anthroposophical practitioners. If so, why?
A. Generally, the medium of art is a very useful activity to learn the art of breathing. Painting is a way of learning how to use the brush and this can be very relaxing. There are many other techniques that assist in getting the rhythmic system to balance the other two systems in the body, such as eurhythmy (a system of training through physical movement to music), hydrotherapy and massage, and all these can be used to help the patient to attain that state of balance.

Q. Is there a specific medication that you would recommend?
A. Gencydo – a preparation based on lemon – is normally used for hay fever and asthma. It has an astringent action on the mucous membranes. The peel of a lemon contains a lot of silica and the acids help the forming and reforming of the boundaries, thus alleviating and guarding against the inflammatory reactions. This preparation is available for direct application as nasal drops, as ointment, or as an injection. Another substance used is copper. It is used in a number of different forms in 'potentised' preparations as it relaxes the smooth muscle and has a warming effect which loosens cramp. These medications are generally used in conjunction with other treatments, such as art therapy, massage and eurhythmy.

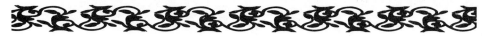

Finding A Practitioner

Anthroposophical practitioners are qualified medical doctors who have then taken a further post-graduate course recognised by the Anthroposophical Medical Association in Britain. Some may be found working in the NHS, although others work privately or in the Rudolf Steiner schools and homes for children. Residential treatment in certain private clinics is also available.

Consultations are very much like seeing a GP except that there will be additional questions, such as about diet, lifestyle and emotional conditions. Practitioners may try and bring about long-term changes, as well as alleviating symptoms, by prescribing eurythmy or an art therapy in order to sort out an underlying imbalance that they think is inherent, and might send a patient to a specialist.

The Anthroposophical Medical Association maintains a register of members. It is based at the Park Attwood Therapeutic Centre, Trimpley, Bewdley, Worcestershire, DY 12 1RE.

Further Reading

Anthroposophical Medicine by Dr. M. Evans and I. Roger (Thorsons).
Anthroposophical Medicine and Its Remedies by Otto Wolf (Weleda Ag).
Rudolf Steiner: Scientist of the Invisible by A.P. Shepherd
  (Floris Books).

7

AROMATHERAPY: NOT JUST AN EXOTIC TREATMENT

Not so long ago, most people would have raised their eyebrows at the very mention of aromatherapy. Today, more and more of us are succumbing to its relaxing benefits – mainly to overcome stress. But aromatherapy can also help asthmatics and those with hay fever.

A New Name For An Ancient Therapy

Aromatherapy uses the healing power of plant essences to alleviate various disorders through the use of essential oils in massage, inhalation, compresses or oral ingestion.

Although the term 'aromatherapy' was not coined until this century, there is much historical evidence to show that the techniques involved were being used as far back as 18,000 BC judging by the dating of paintings on the walls of the Lascaux caves in the Dordogne, France, which show the use of plants in medicine.

The earliest written text to mention the healing powers of scents from plant oils and techniques of using them is Chinese and dates from 1,000–700 BC, while the Egyptians used aromatherapy in embalming, medicine and perfume. Indeed, when Tutankhamun's tomb was opened in 1922, pots containing substances such as myrrh and frankincense, were discovered, and these are known to have been used at the time for such purposes. The Egyptians used aromatic principles in cookery and spices such as coriander and aniseed were added to breads of millet and barley to ease and aid digestion. The Romans, too, used plants in their medicine, and it was the advance of the Roman legions around Europe that contributed to the increase of the types of plants available. Fennel, parsley and lovage are examples of the plants introduced into England by the Romans.

Although the study of natural medicine declined in Europe after its early beginnings, it was actively practised by the Chinese, Indian and Arab peoples. The Arab physician and philosopher Abu Ali Ibn Sina, born 980 AD and known in the West as *Avicenna*, is widely

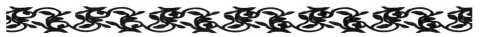

regarded as the inventor of the process of steam distillation as a means of extracting essences from plants, the principles of which are still in use today.

From the Renaissance (the great revival of art, literature and learning in Europe in the fourteenth, fifteenth and sixteenth centuries), there was an upturn in the study of medicine. The colonial explorations, especially the opening up of America to Europe, resulted in a great many new plant species being introduced into Europe. From then on, there was an increase in the manufacture and use of essential oils, which were widely used as antiseptics, perfumes and medicines.

However, chemistry began to flourish as a discipline in the nine-teenth century and this enabled plant cures to be synthesised in a laboratory. These chemical copies took the place that essential oils had traditionally occupied but, although they were cheap to manufacture, the synthetic copies lacked the same medicinal properties as the essential oils.

The twentieth century has seen a renewal of interest in natural treatments, with a consequent demand for genuine essential oils. It was Professor René Gattefosse who pioneered the revival of the use of essential oils in modern medicine. Having accidentally discovered the healing power of the oil of lavender on burns, he went on to research further the effects of essential oils, primarily by using plant essences on wounded soldiers in the First World War. And it was he who coined the word 'aromatherapy'. Gattefosse's work was carried on by the French physician Dr Jean Valnet, who used the essential oils of clove, lemon and chamomile as natural disinfectants and antiseptics to fumigate hospital wards and to sterilise surgical instruments. Marguerite Maury, a French biochemist, extended the research still further by bringing aromatherapy into the spheres of cosmetics and health and beauty.

From trial and error in the earliest days, aromatherapy has developed into a sophisticated and well-researched discipline, taking an important place in modern medicine.

How And Why Does Aromatherapy Work?

Aromatherapy is a fascinating art that involves the use of essential oils in various treatments to facilitate equilibrium not only in physical but also in mental and emotional health. As with the other natural therapies, its nature is holistic. It is also concerned with the

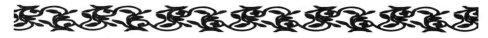

prevention of disease and actively promotes healthy living.

There are two essential components of aromatherapy – the essential oils themselves, which are the 'materials' of the therapy, and their 'method' of administration, such as inhalation, baths, compresses and, most importantly, massage.

Materials

Essential oils are found in plants and herbs, giving fragrance to such flowers as roses and jasmine, or flavour to such herbs as cinnamon and peppermint.

They are extracted from all parts of the plant, from leaves and flowers to roots, seeds and rinds, mostly by the process of steam distillation. Steam is passed under pressure through the plant material. The heat causes the release and evaporation of the oil, which then passes through a water cooler where it condenses and is collected. The average yield of an essential oil from plant substances is 1.5 per cent. Simply put, this means that, on average, 70 kg of plant material is needed to distil just 1 kg of oil. Rose and jasmine are the most expensive essential oils because their yield is relatively tiny.

These aromatic oils are considered to contain the 'life force' of the plants they are extracted from, and are thought to enhance well-being and harmony of mind. Although each particular oil has its own therapeutic properties, they also have powerful antiseptic properties which can destroy bacteria and viruses. They stimulate the immune system, encouraging the body to resist disease, as well as improving the circulation in the body, relieving pain and reducing fluid retention.

Essential oils are chemically very complex substances, and their effect on the human body is similarly complex. They consist of about 100 different chemicals in varying amounts, each constituent, however minor, performing some vital function. This is why synthetic equivalents can never be equally as effective. For example, lemongrass oil has, as its major constituent, an aldehyde, *citral*, which makes up 80 per cent of it. However, if the citral is extracted or synthesised chemically and then applied to the skin, it causes an allergic reaction. Interestingly, lemongrass oil itself does not cause an allergic reaction. Testing has shown that the other 20 per cent of constituents in lemongrass oil can help to neutralise the harmful effects of the citral.

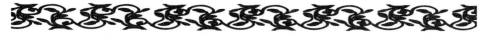

How and why essential oils have a particular effect is not always known scientifically. However, if it works, it works, and is not to be rejected, even if there is no conclusive scientific explanation.

The Importance Of Smell And Touch

In order to understand why aromatherapy is effective, it helps to have a grasp of the way in which our senses of smell and touch work.

As its name suggests, aromatherapy uses aroma, or odour, to create an effect in the human body. Research indicates that our sense of smell works on a subconscious level, and that smell can affect emotional behaviour. Olfactory nerves (those to do with the sense of smell) affect memory. Different odours can arouse the brain and evoke images or feelings associated with that particular smell. Aromatherapy uses this technique in dealing with the mental and emotional aspects of healing. Different smells are used to relax or stimulate the patient, depending on his or her requirements.

Touching is essential for good health. As babies and young children, it is the most important medium through which love is communicated. The use of massage in aromatherapy builds on this. The pleasurable sensation of being touched induces feelings of being loved and cared for.

Massage confers physical as well as emotional benefits on the recipient. The immune system is believed to be stimulated, high blood pressure is reduced and there is improved circulation of the blood and lymph systems. Massage reduces muscular tension or swelling, as well as relieving pain in muscles and joints. This helps the body to relax, which in turn alleviates mental tension and turbulent emotion.

Specific problem areas can also be treated. Some major organs of the body, such as the large intestine, are directly accessible to massage, while other more internally placed organs, such as the liver and kidneys, are influenced by massaging the area of the body where they are situated. This is believed to stimulate the ailing organs by increasing the local blood supply and stimulating the nerves.

Pressure point techniques, so essential to acupressure and reflexology, are used in a more sophisticated massage therapy, when massage with essential oils is concentrated on the pressure points which stimulate specific internal organs.

Other techniques include the use of aromatic baths, which can act either as tonics or sedatives. Hot water opens sores and enables the

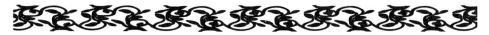

body to absorb essential oils more quickly. Baths can help relieve the effects of stress as well as alleviating muscular pain and skin conditions. Inhalation of essential oils can be effective when the aromatic molecules of essential oils reach the lungs. The molecules diffuse across the air sacs into the capillaries (delicate, thin-walled blood vessels) and find their way into the main blood vessels from where they exercise their therapeutic effect.

Carriers For Essential Oils

- **Air** *for treating colds, headaches and insomnia:* one of the best ways of using pure essential oils is by inhalation where air is the carrier. Put 5 to 10 drops on a tissue and take deep breaths.
- **Water** *to relax:* soaking for 10 minutes in a bath with essential oils is very relaxing and beneficial.
- **Oils** *for massage:* the best known vegetable oils used as carriers are almond, grapeseed and sunflower seed. A few drops of essential oils are added to the carrier oil and massaged into the body.

The Alleviation Of Stress

'Stress' is a term which encompasses a wide spectrum of problems and symptoms which, in turn, can lead to more serious illnesses. Aromatherapy helps to allay the more dangerous conditions caused by stress and is, therefore, preventive in nature. The technique of massage produces in the patient a relaxed and more peaceful state of mind, providing the opportunity to take stock of the problems contributing to stress and to put them in perspective. Pent-up emotions are often released during and after an aromatic massage.

Again, it is the combination of essential oils and massage which is effective – the oils working on the mental tension and the massage alleviating the physical tension. Sleep patterns improve and this leads to a greater feeling of vitality and physical energy.

Stress-related disorders, such as digestive problems, acne and skin problems and headaches, can all be treated. The therapy works in diverse ways, but in part it is due to the release of mood-inducing chemicals in the brain and body, which may act as stimulants or as sedatives. Some essential oils are instrumental in the release of natural painkillers, and there are many conditions involving pain where aromatherapy has been able to help, including, for example,

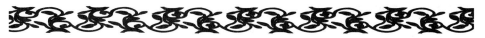

the pain and distress caused by bee and wasp stings, toothache and headaches.

The Treatment

A professional aromatherapy treatment involves a thorough consultation. The therapist will enquire into your personal details, such as age and lifestyle, as well as your general state of health and previous medical history. Diagnosis may take the form of a clinical diagnosis in which the patient may be referred to a doctor, or the form of a holistic diagnosis, which does not identify a specific disease but rather an area of weakness. Holistic diagnostic techniques include muscle testing and foot reflexology. Diagnosis enables the correct essential oils to be chosen for the patient. These are then applied to the body and the face.

Specialised massage movements are used to stimulate the circulation and to activate the lymphatic system. This helps with the removal of toxins from the body. Lymph drainage techniques and pressure points are used. At the end of a session, you are likely to feel a deep sense of well-being and relief from many of the symptoms you have been suffering from.

For asthmatics and hay fever sufferers, a treatment concentrating on the face and pressure points surrounding the sinus cavities has the ability to relieve nasal catarrh.

Self-treatment using aromatic oils is worth considering, too. Keep aromatic oils handy for burns, stings or headaches or for a pleasurable and relaxing bath. However, essential oils should be handled with care as some can be potentially dangerous in the hands of an inexperienced amateur. For serious ailments or for the alleviation of a long-term problem, a professional aromatherapist should always be consulted.

Asthma

Care must be taken when using essential oils for the treatment of asthma. Although oils such as benzoin, eucalyptus or rosemary are commonly used to alleviate respiratory disorders, many leading aromatherapists stress the avoidance of steam inhalations of essential oils by asthma sufferers, warning that concentrated steam may actually trigger an attack.

Instead, other aromatherapy methods of treatment are

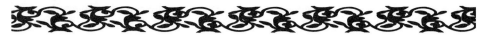

encouraged. Drinking herbal tisanes, for example, made from eucalyptus, thyme, marjoram and savory, can be effective. Fresh rosemary in little pillows situated near a sufferer when sleeping helps to counteract breathing problems.

Chest rubs containing the oils of eucalyptus, juniper or wintergreen are suggested, while oils such as peppermint and rosemary can be inhaled from a tissue when breathing becomes difficult.

Hay Fever

Treatments for hay fever include:

- drinking tisanes made from pine needles and eucalyptus leaves, gargling with lemon juice or boiled water with a drop of tea tree oil
- inhalations containing a few drops of cajeput, eucalyptus, niaouli or tea tree oil
- rubs and handkerchief inhalations of the above-mentioned oils
- itchy eyes can be treated by applying compresses soaked in calendula, chamomile or parsley infusions
- basil is also effective for the loss of sense of smell in hay fever – put one drop of basil oil in a bowl of hot water and inhale 2 to 3 times a day
- infuse 30 ml rose petals in 600 ml boiling water for 10 minutes and gargle

A Conversation With An Aromatherapist

Q. What would the nature of a treatment be for an asthmatic patient?
A. Well, every person is different. I have a particular interest in healing and I tend to work on their stress rather than particular symptoms. Massage itself is very relaxing, so it is something that has a cumulative effect. I'd be a bit concerned about using essential oils though, as they can be allergic.

Q. Does that imply that asthma attacks can be triggered by some essential oils?
A. Yes. I wouldn't want to take that kind of responsibility, but there may be other practitioners that would. For asthma, homoeopathy is best because it can go much deeper and, as for massage, you could do it without having to use essential oils. Additionally, breathing exercises and even yoga could be useful.

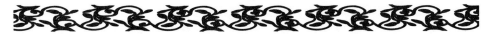

Q. So you seem to advocate an integrated treatment?
A. Yes. Some aromatherapists will use oils in the bath. A popular one is lavender. Some practitioners will use frankincense. I wouldn't say that it's a cure, but frankincense can help deepen breathing and that then helps on a psychological level. The aroma itself is important for the relaxation, and I choose aromas that appeal to people, ones that they have a preference for. There's no point in using oils that they would dislike as they would just tense up. One of the best oils is rose otto but, unfortunately, it's very expensive. It's semi-solid at room temperature. The other rose oil on the market is rose absolute, which is chemically extracted and there may be traces of chemical solvents left in the oil. The rose otto which comes from Bulgaria is fortunately very concentrated, and one drop is usually enough in 25 ml, and you could use that as a chest massage.

Q. How effective are chest rubs of oils, such as eucalyptus, for asthma?
A. Well, I think it's the massage that's effective, especially with clients who suffer from allergies like hay fever. I sometimes teach self-massage techniques that they could use at home. Massage (unfortunately it's not a cure) needs to be done often. I think the two together, the oils and the massage, are much better than the oils on their own.

Q. So with asthma it's better to avoid direct usage of essential oils and steam inhalations.
A. Well, yes. I'm more worried about self-treatment. If well-qualified aromatherapists feel that way inclined, I'm sure they would treat clients in conjunction with natural therapies, like herbal remedies, and not essential oils. My work deals mainly with people suffering from stress. Much of what I do is to help people to relax, which leads on to the alleviation of other problems such as breathing difficulties. Regular massage helps, as does concern for diet and levels of stress.

Q. How would you handle a hay fever case?
A. Again, it's the massage. It helps to relax the whole nervous system. It is mainly stress related. The interesting thing is that many of the hay fever sufferers I've seen seem to be very angry as well. I don't know whether there's any connection. This was the case with my husband, which is why I also give him Bach Flower Remedies. Again, it can't be standardised; it depends on the individual. For example, my husband takes the holly Bach Flower Remedy. He has a weekly massage and takes herbal teas. Eucalyptus is an especially useful oil as he as an allergy to animals. Other useful oils are rose otto, frankincense, and chamomile. As well as inhalation from a few drops on a handkerchief, a daily bath with six

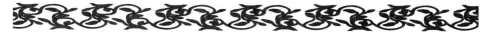

drops of any of the oils and a massage where there is complete relaxation can help.

Q. Is it wise to stick to one oil or opt for a combination in a treatment?
A. It depends. Some oils smell best in combination. For inhalation, a few drops on a handkerchief of just one oil, such as eucalyptus, is sufficient, but oils such as rose and chamomile can be mixed for a massage, or rose, chamomile and frankincense. Again, it may not suit everybody. You have to let people smell the oils individually as, usually, if you're allergic to them you sneeze straightaway. I tend to prefer a low concentration, about 1 drop per 5 ml, so that would be 5 to 6 drops in 25 ml of oil. With allergies it's much better to take it in smaller doses. It also depends on the oils. Chamomile has a very strong odour and usually 2 drops are sufficient in 25 ml of oil.

Q. How do the aromatherapeutic techniques actually help?
A. They work on several levels. The aroma itself is inhaled into the lungs where it has antiseptic qualities . The essential oils also get to the bloodstream as their tiny aromatic molecules diffuse across the alveoli (tiny air sacs in the lungs) and into the bloodstream. It wouldn't be enough to be measured. In addition, oils can be absorbed through the skin.

I think the smell is very important. It's whether you like the aroma. The interesting thing is that if you use rose oil it contains a substance that acts as an opiate, which helps release 'happiness' chemicals so that in itself relaxes the body. The immune system is stimulated. Some oils are 'cooling' and can clear the head.

Q. Do the remedies that you've outlined get to the cause of the problem, or is it more a case of alleviating the symptoms?
A. This is something that has concerned me a lot. In a way, it must be symptomatic. If you use the same oil for too long, it stops working. I think that to get to the root of the problem you can't just use the oils. You have to look at diet and stress levels. I think that it's more than just oils. The oils help, but I think that if you're going to go for a cure I would also then opt for homoeopathy.

Q. So aromatherapy can be integrated with homoeopathy?
A. Well, some say that essential oils can antidote homoeopathy, but what I've found is that the aromatherapy actually prepares the body for homoeopathy. The massage, too, contributes.

I think that the oils alone are symptomatic and alone they cannot be used as cures, but used in combination they are much better at getting to the root of the problem. In any therapy diet is important. If you persist

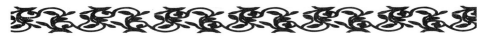

in drinking and smoking, using oils is not going to be that effective. It is important to engage the body and the mind.

Q. If somebody is taking orthodox medication for hay fever, can this be used in conjunction with aromatherapy?
A. I wouldn't actually say to someone that you mustn't take this or that drug. It is difficult, I suppose, because the drugs are so strong they more or less counteract the therapy. Most of the clients I see don't take them, which is why they are trying alternative medicine. I suppose that if the doctor could monitor the patient as they came off the drugs it could help.

Q. Do you find that people come to you as a last resort?
A. Well, some of them do but often, by that time, their bodies are so full of toxins that it's a long haul and they lose patience. With this sort of therapy, it's important to want to help yourself. That's the thing – teaching people to help themselves. It totally depends on the individual how much they are going to take this to heart. Some people just come to aromatherapy for superficial reasons, while there are others that, without being fanatical, look at other ways of relaxing. I teach people to do massage for themselves.

Q. On average, how many sessions would it take for a course of treatment for a condition such as hay fever?
A. Usually, about half a dozen but, gradually, as people do other things, such as look at their diet, visits can be reduced. After the first six or so sessions, people usually come to me for top up. Massage is ongoing. Some people need more sessions depending on their lifestyle and stress levels.

Q. What about self-treatment for hay fever using aromatherapy?
A. Yes, it can be done, but aromatherapy is a complementary therapy so if the hay fever is really bad, I'd recommend homoeopathy.

Q. Where should one look for a practitioner?
A. The best thing to do is to contact the International Federation of Aromatherapists and they would send a list of reputable aromatherapists. Apart from that, it's word of mouth. You can't only go with qualifications. It's an individual thing as you have to get on well with your aromatherapist. It doesn't matter how good you are if there is a clash of personalities.

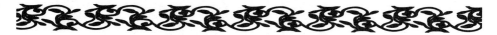

Finding A Practitioner

Aromatherapy Organisations Council, 3 Latymer Close, Braybrooke, Market Harborough, Leicestershire, LE16 8LN.
The International Federation of Aromatherapists, 4 East Mearn Road, Dulwich, London, SE21 8HA, maintains a list of practising aromatherapists.

Further Reading

Aromatherapy – Massage With Essential Oils by Christine (Wildwood Element Books).
Aromatherapy by Daniele Ryman (Piatkus).
Aromatherapy: Headway Lifeguides by Denise Brown (Hodder & Stoughton).
Massage: Headway Lifeguides by Denise Brown (Hodder & Stoughton).
The Art of Aromatherapy by Robert Tisserand (C W Daniels).

8

OTHER TECHNIQUES

Breathing And Stress Control

Breathe in for life, for life is but a series of breaths (a yogic saying)

From the time we take that first gasp at birth and give a shrill wail, we are dependent upon air for our very survival. Breathing is fundamental to life. We can live for weeks without food, but can only last a few minutes without air.

Breathing is a continuous process that provides our lungs with a constant supply of air from which essential oxygen is absorbed into the bloodstream. Breathing out expels unwanted waste as carbon dioxide.

Good breathing, if practised regularly, keeps us calm and helps us to cope with stress. We all experience stress in different ways and in varying degrees. It can be related to work, lifestyle, bereavement, etc. Sometimes, anticipation of an event can cause stress as well. A visit to the dentist or a job interview may give us a sleepless night.

Anticipation of an attack in an asthmatic or a hay fever sufferer can often lead to anxiety and a tightness in the chest, which brings on an attack. Stress can, therefore, become a significant contributory factor, almost like a self-fulfilling prophecy.

Whatever the cause, relaxation is of great therapeutic value. How you relax is up to you. For some, exercising is enough. Others may find one of a variety of relaxation techniques, such as yoga and meditation, helpful.

Correct breathing techniques should be part of an overall asthma management programme – something that seems to have been forgotten in today's over-reliance on drugs.

How To Breathe

There are two basic types of breathing. 'Chest breathing' is the way we quickly get oxygen into the system. It is usually used in times of anxiety, fear or exercise. The chest muscles attached to the ribs

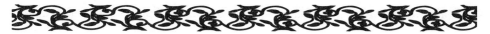

contract, forcing the chest to expand outwards so that air is drawn into the lungs. This type of breathing is fast but shallow, and results in increased muscle tension. While this kind of breathing is necessary, and can even be life saving in certain situations, it can lead to a permanently stressed state for the body if it becomes a regular breathing pattern.

With the frenetic lifestyles so many of us lead, we tend to forget the natural way of breathing which we used instinctively as babies. This is the 'diaphragmatic' manner of breathing. In fact, this is the way we breathe when we are relaxed. Instead of using the chest muscles, breathing occurs by the rhythmic contraction and relaxation of the diaphragm, an umbrella-shaped muscle in the waist area.

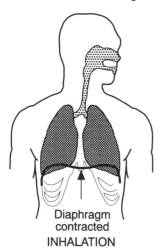

During inhalation the diaphragm moves downwards, thus increasing the space in the chest. This action sucks air into the lungs.

Diaphragm contracted
INHALATION

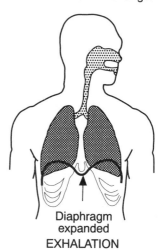

During exhalation the diaphragm moves upwards, thus reducing the space in the chest. This action forces air out of the lungs.

Diaphragm expanded
EXHALATION

The diaphragm flattens to make room as we inhale and domes again as we exhale. This way of breathing is very efficient and promotes relaxation. The lungs are either completely emptied or are filled with breath, so there is little or no build-up of carbon dioxide. It is an indictment on our lifestyles that most of us have to relearn this natural body action because most of us are habitually tense and tend to breathe with our chests. Asthmatics and, for that matter, all of us, could do well to practise diaphragmatic breathing.

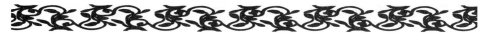

Your first attempt at diaphragmatic breathing will be easier if you lie on your back with a cushion underneath your knees. Rest your hands on your diaphragm, just above the waistline, and breathe in, letting your stomach expand so that your hands rise a little. As you breathe out, your stomach will subside and your hands will go down. Your shoulders should not move at all. With practice it should become easier. For the asthmatic, it is a way of ensuring that every ounce of oxygen is utilised to compensate for a restricted lung capacity.

Yoga can help train the asthmatic to transform laboured breathing into a conscious and positive breathing pattern.

Manipulative Therapies

Osteopathy, chiropractic and the Alexander Technique, among other therapies, can help by teaching us to breathe properly.

Osteopathy

Our bones, joints and muscles form the framework of a complex system that enables us to walk, run, and even sit and lie down. Osteopathy treats mechanical imbalances within that framework in the belief that any abnormality in the system can threaten our health. Maintaining the body in structural balance enables it to heal itself.

Andrew Taylor Still was an American doctor who was influenced by his early training as an engineer. Disenchanted by drug-based medicine, Still studied the interdependence of the various parts of the body structure. Eventually, he was convinced that illness could arise when part of the body was out of alignment. He suggested that manipulation could restore balance and, in turn, cure illness. Further, as a minister's son, he argued that he simply could not believe that God could have created humans without giving them the necessary ability to heal themselves, and that the body contained the secrets of healing.

Still formulated his theory on three very simple principles that came more from conviction than proof:

- the normal, healthy body contains within itself the powers to heal and will deploy its own mechanism of defence and repair of injuries in order to heal itself
- as the body is a unit, an imbalance in one part will inevitably result in an abnormal stress on other parts

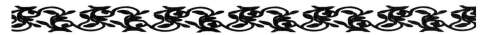

- structural mobility and flexibility are essential for the body to be able to heal itself

In the early days of osteopathy, Still felt that all diseases would respond to his approach. Now with the progress of modern medicine, it is clear that there are better ways of dealing with some of the problems that Still encountered and which the medicine of his time was unable to treat.

Today, osteopaths confine themselves to those problems affecting the bones, joints, muscles and ligaments. Indeed, the bread and butter of most osteopaths' practices are those problems for which GPs are able to offer little more than painkillers. In addition to slipped disks, sciatica, lumbago, fibrositis, trapped nerves or rheumatism, many types of joint or spinal problems are dealt with. Furthermore, osteopathic treatment promotes lymphatic drainage and improves breathing.

In the context of osteopathy, the neck has an important connection with sinus and nasal functions. Displacement of the bones in the upper part of the neck may affect the nerve supply to the respiratory membranes. This displacement is commonly found in people with nasal allergies. Osteopaths explain that the reason why their treatment is conducive to better breathing is because of the important part the spine plays in the breathing process. Asthma is treatable because the restricted rib mobility often found in patients can be improved.

Even a minor displacement in the spine can cause the chest to tighten and breathing to be restricted. Displacements in the chest area mostly affect the ribcage and the part of the spine which supports the ribs. A bad back stance or prolonged coughing can cause pressure on the nerves that affect the chest.

Osteopaths normally work on two levels: the spinal level, because of the spine's direct link to the lungs, including rebalancing of the rest of the body's structure, and the thoracics level, in which they would be helping an asthmatic to breathe out. This is done by manipulating the primary (for example, diaphragm) and secondary (for example, cervical) muscles.

Osteopathic treatment also helps with the elimination of mucus.

Chiropractic

Chiropractors use gentle manipulation to correct disorders of the back joints and of the spine. The most common types of aches and

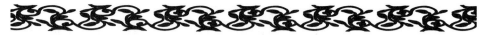

pains they set out to correct are backache, neck pain, low back pain (lumbago), disc lesions, and headache. In many cases, even a migraine headache can be traced to a disturbance of the spine, affecting a part of the nervous system called the *autonomic nervous system* (which functions automatically). Often, disorders of the spine can upset the autonomic nervous system, and various problems that do not seem to be related to the spine can develop, such as dizziness or, in children and young adults, asthma. Occasionally, chiropractic can also relieve other complaints, including catarrh and sinus problems and this can enable an asthmatic to breathe more easily.

The Theory Of Chiropractic

The spinal cord, which passes through the back bones, has nerves radiating off it between the sides of each vertebra. These nerves branch off to the head, trunk, arms and legs. If a vertebra is displaced, this puts pressure on those nerves which, in turn, adversely affects the impulses to the brain and to the rest of the body. It is the job of the chiropractor to discover the misalignment and to manoeuvre the bone back into place, releasing the nerve. The aim is not so much to cure as to enhance the body's own natural healing powers.

During the first consultation, a full case history is taken which includes traumas and injuries going back to childhood, as well as personal habits. A thorough examination is then made which may include the checking of blood pressure, blood tests, and other investigations. X-rays are sometimes used to identify the problem more specifically. Manipulation is the standard procedure, carried out with precision and control, accomplished by quick, light movements.

There are many other techniques which may be used to achieve the chiropractor's aim of better muscle, joint and nerve function. These include sustained pressure on ligaments, stretching of ligaments, and massage of muscles in order to relieve muscle spasm and pain.

The main differences between osteopathy and chiropractic are that osteopaths make more use of the mobilisation of joints and use more 'soft tissue' techniques and greater leverage, while chiropractors employ less leverage and more direct techniques. Contact is made directly over the vertebrae which are being adjusted. Chiropractors also use X-rays seven times more frequently than osteopaths.

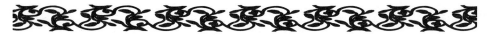

A large majority of qualified chiropractors in the UK belong to the British Chiropractic Association. Practitioners of the McTimoney Technique use one chiropractic technique only, which is claimed to be gentle and sensitive, with the therapist using the intuition of the fingertips for palpation, location and analysis of the relative position of the bones. X-rays are not taken and no diagnosis is made.

Alexander Technique

The Alexander Technique was developed by Frederick Mathias Alexander. It can best be described as a form of re-education, used primarily to rectify faulty habits such as bad posture, bad breathing and speech defects. Secondly, it is a means of helping people to become more aware of themselves and less bound by sheer mechanical habit.

A young actor troubled by voice problems, Alexander found that medical science could do nothing for him. He became convinced that the problem must lie within himself. After years of painstaking research and self-observation, he discovered that while reciting he tended to stiffen his neck and pull his head back and down, thereby depressing his vocal cords and shortening his spine. When he tried to correct this posture directly by putting his head forward, he found he was pressing down on his vocal cords in a different way. The correct posture, he found, could only be achieved by consciously allowing his head to assume its correct orientation in relation to the neck and torso. The Alexander Technique helps to improve posture, resulting in the improvement of health and mental alertness.

It is said that Alexander himself suffered from acute asthma before he discovered the technique. When he started teaching his technique to others, he was called the 'Breathing Man', not just because his own breathing was so well co-ordinated, but because he emphasised retraining in breathing techniques.

Of the many aspects of the technique, those that are most helpful to asthmatics are connected with relaxation and deep breathing. Alexander stressed that if we stopped breathing in the incorrect manner, the right way of breathing would automatically manifest itself. Alexander teachers work with their 'pupils' to effect an improvement in their breathing mechanism.

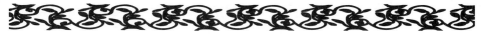

What Does An Alexander Technique Teacher Do?

Most 'pupils', as they are called, rather than patients, are unaware that they have a lot of tension in their chests. Alexander Technique can help by making them aware of this tension and their breathing. After a normal course of three lessons they begin to correct their breathing. The attacks become less frequent and less severe once breathing improves.

Registered teachers belong to the Society of Teachers of the Alexander Technique (STAT), 20 London House, 266 Fulham Road, London, SW10 9EL.

Reflexology

Reflexology is not to be treated lightly as being an 'airy-fairy', 'toe-tickling' therapy. It is, in fact, a serious alternative therapy which is complex and structured. It adopts a holistic approach, aiming to cure not only the symptoms of a particular disease, but also to treat the underlying problem of which the disease might be a symptom.

Reflexology Through The Ages

The technique of using the feet as a barometer of bodily health and as a way of healing has been practised from early times. The origins of reflexology date back at least 5,000 years, and traditional Chinese medicine has always used massage of the feet, hands and body as a basic technique to affect internal organs and muscles. The ancient Egyptians were also known to have been using similar methods. This can be seen from ancient tomb drawings in which feet are being held and massaged. Even in more recent times, it has emerged that some of the Red Indian tribes and tribal peoples of Africa use a form of reflexology.

More 'modern' techniques of reflexology, sometimes known as *zone therapy*, were applied and practised by the American physician Dr William Fitzgerald, working in 1913, who was intrigued by the observation that on some patients he was able to carry out operations on the throat and nose without their feeling any pain yet, on a different patient, a similar operation involved the person being in a considerable amount of pain. On investigation, he found that in those cases where little pain had been experienced the patient had been applying pressure to certain parts of the hand or, perhaps

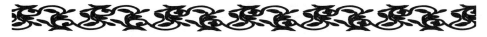

prior to the operation, he himself had applied pressure to certain areas of the body and this had subsequently inhibited pain in other areas. Indeed, subconsciously, we use the basic principles of zone therapy in our lives every day as an automatic response to pain. When we grind or bite on our teeth to reduce pain or rub our hands in an effort to alleviate hurt, this may be a way of putting pressure on those zones in the hand that may reduce pain elsewhere.

These initial findings were tentatively received by the medical profession, although osteopaths and naturopaths were more welcoming. However in the 1940s, some doctors did take an interest. Dr Joe Riley investigated the method extensively, and a protégé of his, Eunice Ingham, pioneered the 'Ingham Compression Method of Reflexology', which concentrated on the reflexes to be found on the feet with massage to be applied to the foot digits as well as the soles and tops of the feet. In her turn, Ingham had a great influence on Mrs Doreen Bayly, and it was she who was primarily responsible for introducing the techniques of reflexology into Britain.

Reflexology has developed from the general principles of zone therapy, in which it was ascertained that certain points on the body influence other parts which are seemingly unconnected, to the specific use of the feet, which are known to be sensitive and receptive to this type of pressurised massage. A reflexologist may occasionally use the hands, but generally the points on the feet are preferred.

The Foot As A Mirror Of The Human Body

The phrase 'zone therapy' gives an indication of the theory behind reflexology. It has emerged, through the research of Dr Fitzgerald and others, that a map of the body can be seen on the soles of the feet. This means that there are points or zones on the foot that correspond to a particular organ or region of the body.

More specifically, ten body zones pass down the body, from the head down to the toes, through all the organs of that zone, and spread out to end in the feet. This is how each important organ or muscle is connected to a particular spot on the foot. Additionally, the organs on the left side of the body connect to the left foot and those on the right to the right foot. The toes and upper part of the feet relate to the head, neck and brain areas, while the points for the lower regions of the body, such as the coccyx or knees, are situated towards the heel of the foot.

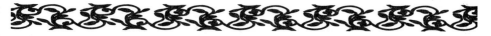

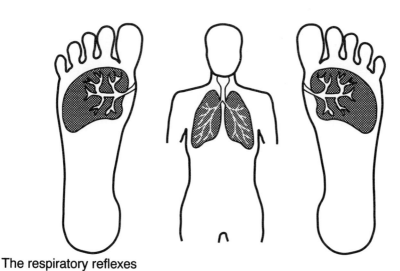

The respiratory reflexes

The theory behind reflexology is that the body's bioelectrical energy flows longitudinally through these zones to the reflex points in the feet and hands and that the obstruction or blocking of this energy is what contributes to ill health. The relationship between any organ or part of the body is such that if there is a problem with any part of the body the corresponding region of the foot will be affected, too.

How Does It Work?

By means of Kirlian photography, which is able to show the energy fields surrounding objects, it has been shown that the energy field present around the reflex in the foot is diminished when there is a problem in the body area corresponding to that reflex area. On treatment, the energy field improves, indicating that it has been successfully balanced.

Gentle pressure on the reflex points will detect pain and small lumps consisting of toxic wastes and unused calcium. It is thought that these small deposits impede the free flow of energy along the zone.

Treatment consists of massaging and moving the foot, thereby dispersing the lumps which are then absorbed into the bloodstream and later expelled from the body in sweat and urine. The body is getting rid of wastes.

The exact scientific explanations for the system are not known, but

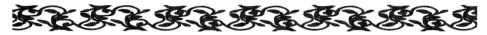

it is evident that reflex massage can dilate or constrict the blood vessels, and can sedate or stimulate pain in areas that are remote from the part that is being massaged. The principle, which is similar to acupressure or acupuncture, is that relaxing or stimulating the body can help sluggish glands and organs return to normal functioning. Reflexology can also help to reduce pain, and it is thought that this is because massaging the reflex areas causes the release of substances, known as *endorphins,* which act as the body's own pain-killing agents.

Applications

The therapy is more useful for simple acute conditions, such as a cold, and for functional disorders, such as constipation or sinus troubles, than for long-term serious medical complaints or emergencies. Headaches can be relieved temporarily by massaging the appropriate points, and the pleasurable sensation of massage aids relaxation and relieves stressful emotions.

Reflexology can also be used as a method of diagnosis. If there is a problem in a specific area, the corresponding reflex point in the foot, when massaged, should elicit pain or show evidence of toxic build-up. However, these points can only indicate that there may be a disorder in the probable organs, not what the disorder is and how serious it may be.

Reflexology is not so much a therapy that cures, although it may effect a cure. Rather it encourages the body to heal itself by stimulating previously sluggish bodily functions and expelling wastes. Seen in this light, reflexology is a preventive therapy which may forestall the development of more serious disorders by encouraging general good health and efficient bodily function. Indeed, many reflexologists claim that potential problems can be picked up early by spotting warning signs in the feet, and relating them to the parts of the body affected.

The Reflexologist

A visit to the reflexologist is recommended if there is a specific problem area. It is common for the therapist to ask the patient personal details, as well as taking a medical history and lifestyle profile.

The session starts off with a massage during which the reflexologist, using the thumb to apply pressure, will go over the feet

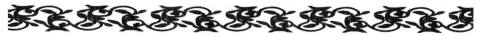

pressing on the points and enquiring whether any pain was felt. The therapist looks for any crystal deposits at the points which will indicate where there might be a problem. If there is a specific complaint, the therapist will usually go over the entire foot and then concentrate on those points which relate particularly to the problem area. The therapist usually uses the hands and, specifically, the thumb, in the massage, although some use a comb or an elbow. Six to eight 1-hour sessions are usually necessary for a treatment programme, although subsequent one-off treatments usually follow.

Asthma And Hay Fever

In treating such conditions, the reflexologist will naturally concentrate on those areas of the feet that correspond to the regions of the body affecting and affected by asthma or hay fever. In both cases, there are direct reflex areas and also associated reflex areas which are specifically massaged.

Asthma

The direct reflex areas which would primarily be treated are the points relating to the lungs and the bronchi. In association, the reflexologist will apply massage to the points relating to the solar plexus, the cervical and thoracic spine, the adrenal glands, the ileo-caecal valve, the pituitary gland, thyroid and reproductive glands, and the heart.

Hay Fever

Massage will be applied to the direct reflex areas corresponding to the sinuses and the eyes. The treatment may also extend to the associated areas of the ileo-caecal valve, the adrenal glands, the spleen and upper lymphatics.

Acupuncture

This therapy, which has its roots in China, has only recently been accepted as an effective means of dealing with a wide variety of illnesses. But now it is frequently used, not just by complementary medical therapists, but also by some orthodox medical practitioners.

It is a technique in which very fine needles are used to puncture

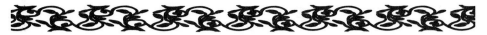

the skin at defined points along the body so as to stimulate and unblock the flow of *chi* energy which acupuncturists believe is essential for good health.

There is no lack of mythical explanations about the origins of acupuncture. Legend has it that this therapy was discovered some 4,000 years ago when it was observed that warriors who were wounded with arrows often recovered from diseases that had troubled them for many years. This is supposed to have sparked off the notion that certain points on the skin correspond to certain functions in the body. Chinese doctors and physicians of the time started experimenting with needles made of stone quarried from rich jade deposits in the mountains of China. Later on, bone and bamboo were used. When metal was discovered, the needles were made of iron, silver, copper, gold and other alloys. Today's needles are made of processed stainless steel and vary from half to one-and-a-half inches in length.

It would appear that over many years, a cause-and-effect relationship was worked out by observant physicians between the point punctured and the disease it cured. Over time, these points were charted and the healing art of acupuncture became established.

The original text that establishes the basis of this system of medicine is *Huang Di Nei Jing*, meaning *The Yellow Emperor's Classic of Internal Medicine*, written some 2,000 years ago.

The Theory And Philosophy

Some knowledge of the philosophical and theoretical bases of this system of medicine is essential for understanding how the therapy works.

The ancient Chinese had a very different view of the cosmos. Very simply, all things are believed to have two aspects – a *yin* aspect and a *yang* aspect. Without these two complementary, yet opposite, parts nothing could exist. It is like saying 'without day there can be no night' and 'without cold there can be no heat'.

Originally, *yin* was understood to encompass all the qualities found on the shady side of a mountain, such as cold, wetness and darkness, and *yang* had the qualities of the sunny side, such as heat, dryness and brightness.

It is also believed that all living matter is permeated by a life force or vital energy, which the Chinese call *chi*. In the human body, *chi* is said to flow along specific pathways called *meridians*. When the body is in a state

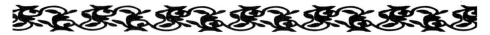

of health, the *yin/yang* aspects of the body's *chi* are in balance, and the body's energies can flow freely. If, however, the *yin/yang* balance of the body is upset, the flow of chi is disturbed, resulting in disease.

From this it is clear that the basis of acupuncture theory is that the root cause of all disease is a disturbance in the energy equilibrium of the body, and that treatment should be directed primarily at restoring the lost equilibrium.

One way of entering into the body's energy network is via the acupuncture points, which are located within the meridians. There are around 800 points on the body, which join up to form 12 major meridians. These meridians (except for the *triple warmer*) are named after the organs to which they are attached: *large intestine; stomach; heart; spleen; small intestine; bladder; circulation; kidney; gall bladder; lung; liver,* plus the two central and governing meridians. By manipulating the points, one can actually influence the *chi* and *yin/yang* balance of the body.

How and Why Does Acupuncture Work?

The fact is, Western scientific approaches to medicine cannot explain acupuncture. One theory is that it assists the body to release the natural painkillers, *endorphins* and *enkephalins.* These complex biochemicals have been known to be beneficial in cases of depression and in allergies. Acupuncture has been shown to increase the levels of endorphins and enkephalins .

Some sceptics attribute to it the 'placebo effect', that simply believing a therapy is effective helps the body to activate its own healing mechanism, but this does not explain the long tradition of veterinary acupuncture. Another idea that has gained currency, especially among Western researchers is the 'gate control theory'. Put simply, pain messages follow paths through the spinal cord to the brain. Acupuncture is supposed to close the gates, thus blocking the pain message to the brain, so that pain subsides, but again, this is only one part of the picture; it does not explain why acupuncture can heal non-painful conditions.

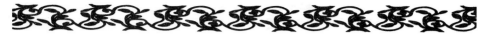

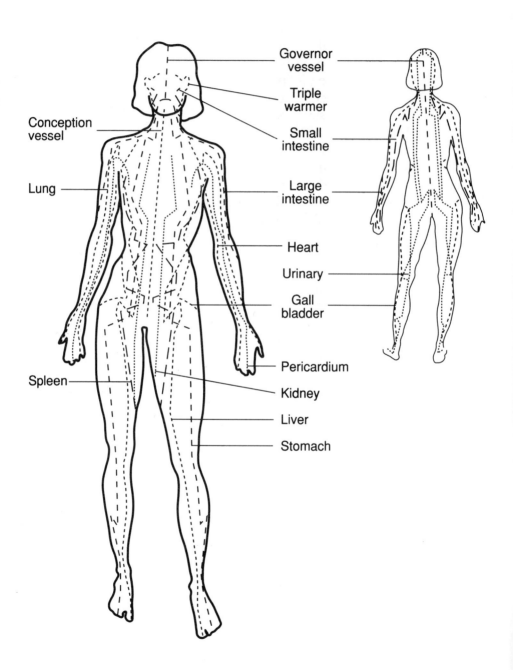

The meridians

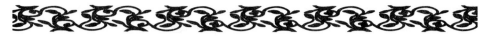

How Does The Acupuncturist Diagnose?

In order to diagnose the nature of the patient's disorder, the acupuncturist will take a full medical history and observe particular features, such as the quality and texture of the skin, the appearance and colour of the face, tongue (in itself a highly refined diagnostic procedure) and eyes, the distinctive odour of the body, and personal gestures and tone of voice. These help him or her to build up a complete picture. A physical examination may follow, depending on the practitioner.

The next procedure is to check the pulses, of which there are 12, one for each meridian, six to each wrist. There are 28 qualities which can be ascertained from the pulses, for example, tight, hasty, thin, weak, long, fine, slow. Refinement of this technique takes many years, and by mastering it the acupuncturist gains an insight into the seriousness of the disorder and how to treat it.

There is an interesting story about the use of the pulse diagnosis in ancient China. Women of royalty were not allowed to be seen by their physician and the only method available to the doctor was pulse analysis. The physician and the patient were separated by a veil or curtain, and the patient would slide her hand under this protective barrier and the acupuncturist was able to take her pulses. Simply on this basis alone, the practitioners were known to have made remarkably accurate diagnoses of the particular ailments.

Having made a diagnosis, the acupuncturist then decides which acupuncture points to focus on in order to restore the balance in the patient's energy pattern. Each point has a particular function attributed to it, and this determines which points need to be stimulated. The most common way to stimulate acupuncture points is with needles.

Why Needles?

Many people hate the thought of needles as they have unpleasant connotations. But according to those who undergo acupuncture, it is a relatively painless process. Insertion by a skilled practitioner feels somewhat like a small pinprick followed by a feeling of tingling, fullness or pressure, which may be felt up to half an hour after treatment. When done correctly, it draws no blood.

To restore *chi* energy, the needles may be inserted obliquely, vertically or almost horizontally. Sometimes they just penetrate the skin, or they can be sunk to a depth of an inch or more. They may

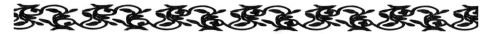

then be twirled or slightly lifted or thrusted to summon the energy. Needles may be left in place for a few seconds or up to a period of one hour, depending on the situation.

Some acupuncturists attach a mild electric current to the needles. They claim it regulates the energy flow with more precision. This is mostly for analgesia. This technique is called *electro-acupuncture*, but this is not a part of acupuncture practice.

Pain Relief

Acupuncture can be used to relieve pain, especially chronic pain, without the side-effects of drugs. It can also be used as an anaesthetic during operations. This was first tried in 1958 when a patient underwent an operation to remove his tonsils with only the needles acting as anaesthetic. The patient reported no pain and no after-effects. A year later, it was successfully used in surgery of the brain, chest, limbs, abdomen and back. Today, more than a million doctors in China rely solely on it as an anaesthetic during surgery.

A form of acupuncture that relies solely on the ear is called *auriculotherapy*. It bases its treatment on the correlation between the ear and other parts of the body, recognising in the structure of the ear a mirror image of the human foetus in its intra-uterine position – inverted with the head pointing downwards. Two hundred points have been found on the ear. Treatment is usually carried out by an electronic instrument that detects the points and simultaneously stimulates them, although often needles are used, as an adjunct to 'body' acupuncture.

Because traditional Chinese medicine treats the individual as a whole person, rather than specific symptoms, it can help most ailments. However, there is no such thing as an instant cure because disease has to work its way out of the body. A long-standing illness may take considerably longer to do this than one recently contracted.

Hay Fever

In traditional Chinese medicine, hay fever is regarded as a yang condition caused by the rising of 'fire' from the liver and gall bladder. To disperse the heat and congestion, needles may be inserted on the face and the forehead. The large intestine meridian, which runs up from the back of the hand over the side of the elbow on to the neck and terminates after crossing the midline at the side

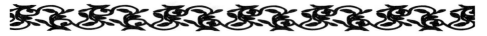

of the nose, is the one on which lie an important chain of points for treating hay fever and other ear, nose and throat conditions. Treatment takes place using the points on this channel both locally, around the nose and upper lip, and on the tops of the hands. This clears the nasal passages and reduces inflammation. A brief course of acupuncture in early spring is all that is needed.

Integrated Treatment

According to Dr William Khoe, there was a 90 per cent success rate in the treatment of 500 cases of hay fever and rhinitis using a combination of acupuncture, homoeopathy and nutrition.

Finding An Acupuncturist

Anyone can use the title 'acupuncturist', which makes it all the more important that you ensure that the practitioner is properly trained. There are four professional bodies which are affiliated to the Council for Acupuncture, 38 Mount Pleasant, London WC1X OAP, which maintains a register of practitioners. They are the British Acupuncture Association and Register, the International Register of Oriental Medicine UK, the Register of Traditional Chinese Medicine, and the Traditional Medicine Society. Before qualifying, students have to undergo a minimum three-year course which includes subjects such as anatomy, diagnosis, pathology and physiology.

Acupressure

The Chinese discovered the healing and health-maintaining effects of acupressure more than 5,000 years ago. Acupressure is a combination of the techniques of acupuncture and massage: similar to acupuncture in that it uses the same points, dissimilar in that massage techniques are used in place of needles.

When you have a headache and rub your temples, you are employing acupressure to relieve the pain. Similarly, when you knock your elbow, for example, and rub it to ease the pain, that is also acupressure. Acupressure is the art of using the fingers to press particular points (the acupuncture points) on the body to stimulate the body's own healing powers. It can be practised anytime, anywhere and by yourself. The only equipment needed are your

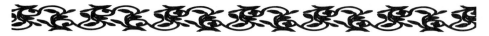

own two hands. Tension, stress and insomnia are only some of the health problems which can be improved with acupressure.

How it works

Although there are various kinds of acupressure, all use the same pressure points, described as *potent points*. The potent points are the same as those identified in acupuncture, occurring on the 12 meridians through which *chi*, the body energy, passes. Stimulation of the potent points with needles, as in acupuncture, or finger or heat pressure with acupressure, releases *endorphins*; these are the body's natural painkillers. When endorphins are released in the body, pain sensation is blocked and oxygen flow increases. This in turn relaxes the muscles and promotes healing.

The potent points, by their very nature, tend to accumulate tension. Fatigue, stress, trauma and chemical imbalance prompt secretion of lactic acid. This in turn causes the muscles to contract and tense up. Pressure applied to a potent point stretches the muscle fibres; this improves blood circulation and enables the body to eliminate toxins. This, of course, is beneficial to the immune system and as a result increases the body's resistance to illnesses.

Finding the Potent Points

There are three types of points: local, trigger and tonic.
Local Point: this is the actual place where pain is felt. Stimulation of a point in the same area as the pain itself brings relief.
Trigger Point: a local point can also trigger an effect in another part of the body which is on the same meridian.
Tonic Point: these are points which maintain general good health. A popular tonic point is the webbing between the thumb and index finger.

The points each have two methods of identification. There is the original ancient Chinese name, which often describes the healing benefit. For example, *Shoulder Corner* describes the point to ease shoulder pain; *Three Mile Point* is so called because it apparently gives enough energy to run three miles! Chanting the name of a point whilst putting pressure on it is said to aid meditation and encourage 'mind over body' healing. In addition, each point has a modern classification consisting of letters and numbers. This classifications is universally used by professional practitioners both of acupressure

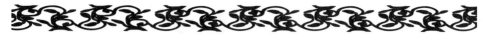

and acupuncture. The points can be located by reference to anatomical pointers such as bone indentations and other organs.

How to practise acupressure

There are four main types of pressure: firm, slow, brisk rubbing and quick tapping.

Thumbs, fingers, the palm of the hand and the knuckles are used to apply firm pressure. Areas of the body which have the more developed muscles, for example the shoulder and buttocks, need firm pressure. Pressure is applied for several minutes to relax an area or to relieve pain, for a few seconds if the intention is simply to stimulate circulation.

Slow, kneading movements are used to loosen up stiff muscles. Brisk rubbing increases circulation, tones the skin and relieves chills and numbness.

Quick tapping with the fingertips is for tender areas, such as the face, and improves nerve functioning.

Ideally, you should practise acupressure on a daily basis, for an hour at the most, but two or three times a week will also net benefits.

Relieving Breathing Difficulties

The point associated with the lung (*B13*) is located just below the upper tip of the shoulder blade and and the spine. Press this point with your finger, first on your right side and then the left, while taking deep breaths.

The other useful pair points associated with relieving asthma, named the *Elegant Mansion* point (*K27*), are located in the indentation directly below the collar bone. Apply firm pressure as you take deep breaths.

A Visit to an Acupressure Practitioner

Acupressure can be practised by yourself, but a course in the technique by a professional is useful. Practitioners will usually use firm thumb or fingertips to massage on the potent points, although elbows and even knees may be used. Sessions typically last between 30 and 60 minutes.

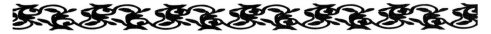

Finding A Practitioner

The General Council and Register of Osteopaths, 56 London Street, Reading, Berkshire, RG14BQ.

The British Naturopathy and Osteopathy Association, 6 Netherall Gardens, London, NW3 5RR.

The British Chiropractic Association, 29 Whitley Street, Reading, Berkshire, RG2 2EG.

The Institute of Pure Chiropractic, 14 Park End Street, Oxford OX2 1HH.

Society of Teachers of the Alexander Technique (STAT), 10 Station House, 266 Fulham Road, London, SW10 9EL.

The Council for Acupuncture, 38 Mount Pleasant, London, WC1X OAP.

The British Reflexology Association, 12 Pond Road, London, SE3 9JL, maintains a register of members which is updated three times a year. Its official teaching body is the Bayley School of Reflexology.

Further reading

Acupuncture by Alexander Macdonald (George Allen & Unwin)
Acupressure's Potent Points by Michael Reed Gach (Bantam Books)
Alexander Technique: Headway Lifeguides by Glynn Macdonald
  (Hodder & Stoughton)
Art of Changing - A New Approach to The Alexander Technique
  by Glen Park, (Ashgrove Press)
Chiropractic by S. Moore (Macdonald Optima)
Chiropractic Today by Copland-Griffiths (Thorsons)
Osteopathy Self Treatment by Leon Chaitow (Thorsons)
Reflexology & Colour Therapy Workbook by Pauline Wills
  (Element Books)
Reflexology: Headway Lifeguides by Chris Stormer
  (Hodder & Stoughton)
The Alexander Technique - Natural Poise For Health by Richard Brennan,
  (Element Books)

9

CONCLUSION

The thirteenth century Persian poet and mystic, Rumi, once told a story about an elephant in a dark house. As people went to see it all they could do was feel a part of the elephant with their palms. The hand of one fell on the trunk and he said, 'This creature is like a water pipe'. Another laid his hand on the back and said, 'Truly this creature is like a throne'. Yet another found the creature 'Like a pillar', for he had touched the leg. The explanations were limited by what the palm could feel. This is like viewing a human being as a machine and attempting to restore health by repairing the various parts individually.

Among the many scientists and thinkers who have guided modern man is René Descartes, whose dictum, 'I think therefore I am', crystallised the notion of the Cartesian dualism of *res cognitas* (the realm of the mind) and *res extensa* (the realm of matter). In the light of this, the material world came to be viewed as an elaborate machine made of assembled parts. Of the human body Descartes wrote, 'I consider the human body as a machine. My thought compares the sick man and an ill-made clock with my idea of a healthy man and a well-made clock.' This legacy of 'reductionism' has guided and moulded the basis of scientific enquiry up to the present time.

Indeed, the study of disease has focused on biological processes, attributing the causes of all illness to biological factors. Modern medicine, preoccupied with measurements, statistical models and double-blind crossover studies, fails to take into account the person as a whole and appears to preclude the human potential for self-healing. So much has been studied about the 'trunk' or the 'legs' or the 'back' that the elephant has almost been forgotten.

Statistics (another vagary where the patient is a number and the disease an entry) show that, despite massive investment in health care, the level of diseases is rising rapidly. Measured on the yardstick of health, the technological and chemical management of disease reflects a rather sorry state of affairs. The Director General of the World Health Organisation lamented that:

'Most of the world's medical schools produce doctors, not to take care of the health of people but, instead, for a medical practice that is blind to anything

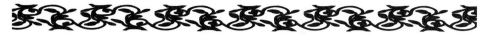

but disease and the technology of dealing with it; a technology involving astronomical and ever-increasing prices directed towards fewer and fewer people ...'

Today, there is no dearth of alternatives to the practice of modern medicine. Indeed, many use traditional methods of treatment which have existed for centuries in such countries as China, India and Japan. Their popularity, however, is largely as a result of disenchantment with the high-tech, high-cost, drug-based orthodox medicine.

In recent years, the holistic model of health care has begun to gain momentum. The proponents of this model have gone some way to counter the mechanistic and reductionist streaks in modern medicine. Holism is based on the premise that the human organism is a multidimensional being, possessing body, mind and spirit, all inextricably linked, and that disease results from an imbalance either from within or from an external force. The human body possesses a powerful and innate capacity to heal itself by bringing itself back into a state of balance and so the primary task of the practitioner is to encourage and assist the body in its attempts to heal itself. The practitioner's role is that of an educator rather than as an interventionist. If the patient sees him or herself as a self-healing agent, he or she will naturally want to exercise his or her own power and to be in control of his or her own health.

This is a dilemma for modern medicine. The issue at stake is who should decide what is best for the patient, who should be 'in charge'? There is a valid argument that it is not possible, or even prudent, to give that power to those who are unable to handle it. In any event, how can a doctor with his or her regulation seven minutes per patient even contemplate being an educator?

Such questions and paradoxes reflect the truncated value system that has dogged us here in the West, and is rapidly disrupting the peoples of the East.

The true test of healing must surely be a practical manifestation of harmony between the mind, the body and spirit. Holism has some answers, but matters of the spirit, while acknowledged, remain untouched and are even avoided in practice. Yet without the spiritual dimension, no system of healing can be truly whole.

The East has taught the West that there are other approaches to health care than that of modern medicine. These disciplines, based on different world views and cosmological principles, all have a common thread – their origin is seen to be divine. It is not enough

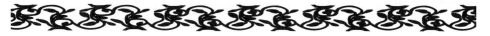

just to learn the techniques. The proponents of holistic medicine must attempt a closer study of the means developed to deal with illness by considering man in the context of his relationship with the cosmos. Can acupuncture, for example, really make sense without the Chinese world view? No wonder we are confused by it. Similarly, holistic medicine will only make sense when it is set within the framework of a world view which gives it the much-needed spiritual dimension.

The Cartesian legacy of dualism and its by-product of reductionism has helped to destroy the concept of the divine here in the West. The cries of holism are a manifestation of our dissatisfaction with the present model. But while it cannot bring the divine back into the system, it can act as a catalyst for future change. Meanwhile, our best bet is the concept of an integrated system in which orthodox medical practitioners join hands with complementary therapists to offer the least imperfect system that such an integration may bring.

We may not be able to see the whole elephant, but let us at least accept that our perception of the elephant is far from complete, and is only limited to the comprehension of the 'palm'.

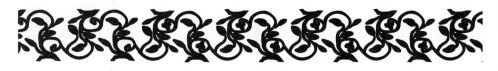

GLOSSARY

Acute Symptom that comes on suddenly, usually for a short period.

Adrenaline Hormone released by the adrenal gland, triggered by fear or stress, also called *epinephrine.*

Allergy A condition caused by the reaction of the immune system to a specific substance.

Allopathy A term used to describe conventional drug-based medicine.

Amino acids A group of chemical compounds containing nitrogen that form the basic building blocks in the production of protein. Of the 22 known amino acids, 8 are considered essential because they cannot be made by the body and therefore must be obtained from the diet.

Anaemia A condition that results when there is a low level of red blood cells.

Analgesic A substance that relieves pain.

Antibiotic A medication that helps to treat infection caused by bacteria.

Antibody Protein molecule released by the body's immune system that neutralises or counteracts foreign organisms *(antigen).*

Antidote A substance that neutralizes or counteracts the effects of a poison.

Antigen Any substance that can trigger the immune system to release an antibody to defend the body against infection and disease. When harmless substances like pollen are mistaken for harmful antigens by the immune system, allergy results.

Antihistamine A chemical that counteracts the effects of histamine, a chemical released during allergic reactions.

Antioxidants Substances which inhibit oxidation by destroying free radicals. Common antioxidants are vitamins A, C, E and the minerals selenium and zinc.

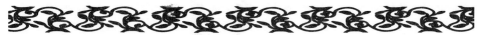

Antiseptic   A preparation which has the ability to destroy undesirable microorganisms.

Artherosclerosis   A disorder caused when fats are deposited in the lining of the artery wall.

Atopy   A predisposition to various allergic conditions like asthma, hay fever, urticaria and eczema.

Auto-immune disease   A condition in which the immune system attacks the body's own tissue e.g. rheumatoid arthritis.

Benign   Non-cancerous cells; not malignant.

Beta carotene   A plant substance which can be converted into vitamin A.

Bile   Liquid produced in the liver for fat digestion.

Candida albicans   Yeast-like fungi found in the mucous membranes of the body.

Carcinogen   Cancer-causing substance or agent.

Cartilage   Connective tissue that forms part of the skeletal system, such as the joints.

Chi   Chinese term for the energy that circulates through the meridians.

Cholesterol   A fat compound, manufactured in the body, that facilitates the transportation of fat in the blood stream.

Chronic   A disorder that persists for a long time; in contrast to acute.

Cirrhosis   Liver disease caused by damage of the cells and internal scarring *(fibrosis)*.

Collagen   Main component of the connective tissue.

Constitutional treatment   Treatment determined by an assessment of a person's physical, mental and emotional states.

Contagious   A term referring to a disease that can be transferred from one person to another by direct contact.

Corticosteroid   Drugs used to treat inflammation similar to corticosteroid hormones produced by the adrenal glands that control the body's use of nutrients and excretion of salts and water in urine.

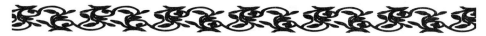

Detoxification   Treatment to eliminate or reduce poisonous substances *(toxins)* from the body.

Diuretic   Substance that increases urine flow.

DNA   A molecule carrying genetic information in most organisms.

Elimination diet   A diet which eliminates allergic foods.

Endorphins   Substances which have the property of suppressing pain. They are also involved in controlling the body's response to stress.

Enzyme   A protein catalyst that speeds chemical reactions in the body.

Essential fatty acids   Substances that cannot be made by the body and therefore need to be obtained from the diet.

Free radicals   Highly unstable atom or group of atoms that can bind to and

Hepatic   Pertaining to the liver.

Histamine   A chemical released during an allergic reaction, responsible for redness and swelling that occur in inflammation.

Holistic medicine   Any form of therapy aimed at treating the whole person – mind, body and spirit.

Iridology   The science of diagnosis by observing the iris of the eye.

Keratin   A protein found in the outermost layer of the skin, nails and hair.

Lymphocyte   A type of white blood cell found in lymph nodes. Some lymphocytes are important in the immune system.

Malignant   A term that describes a condition that gets progressively worse resulting in death.

Melanoma, malignant   A form of skin cancer.

Mast cell   A cell that secretes histamine and other inflammatory chemicals and plays an important part in allergy.

Meridian   Energy pathways that connect the acupuncture and acupressure points and the internal organs.

Mucous membrane   Pink tissue that lines most cavities and tubes in the body, such as the mouth, nose etc.

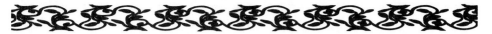

Mucus The thick fluid secreted by the mucous membranes.

Nebuliser An instrument used to apply liquid in the form of fine spray.

Neurotransmitter A chemical that transmits nerve impulses between nerve cells.

Oxidation Chemical process of combining with oxygen or of removing hydrogen.

Placebo A chemically inactive substance given instead of a drug, often used to compare the efficacy of medicines in clinical trials.

Potency A term used in homoeopathy to describe the number of times a substance has been diluted.

Prostaglandin Hormone-like compounds manufactured from essential fatty acids.

Sclerosis Process of hardening or scarring.

Stimulant A substance that increases energy.

Toxin A poisonous protein produced by disease-causing bacteria.

Vaccine A preparation given to induce immunity against a specific infectious disease.

Vasoconstriction A term used to describe the constriction of blood vessels.

Vitamin Essential nutrient that the body needs to act as a catalyst in normal processes of the body.

Withdrawal Termination of a habit-forming substance.

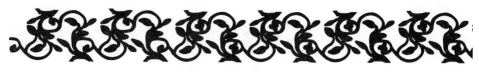

INDEX

Acquired immunity 44
Acupressure 109-111
Acupuncture 103-109
Acute attack 40
Alexander Technique
    98-99
Alkaline foods 41
Allergic response 26
Allergic rhinitis 16
Allergic salute 26
Allergic shiners 26
Allergy 17
Allopathic medicine 57
Anabolic medicine 76-81
Anthroposophical
    medicine 74
Anti-allergic 3.8
Anti-allergy drugs 27
Anti-histamines 24, 27,
    38, 47
Antinutrients 52
Antioxidants 45, 46, 47,
    48, 49, 51
Antiseptics 83, 84
Arachidonic 41
Aromatherapy 82-92
Aromatic baths 85
Aromatic massage 86
Artificial sweeteners 42
Artistic therapies 77
Asthma attack 20
Asthma in children 19,
    31, 34
Atopic 26, 30, 33
Auriculotherapy 108
Autoinhaler 38

Bach Flower
    Remedies 89
Beta carotene 48
Blood purifiers 57

Bronchial asthma 19
Bronchodilator 24, 30,
    36, 40

Cardiac asthma 19
Catabolic 76
Catarrh 42, 58, 97
Chest breathing 93
Chi 65, 104, 107
Chiropractic 96-98
Compresses 84
Corticosteroids 37, 40
Corticosteroid
    hormones 47

Dander 31
Decongestants 29
Demulcents 57
Dependency 63
Desensitisation 29
Diaphragmatic
    breathing 94
Dilutions 66
Diuretics 57
Dry powder inhalers 39

Eczema 19, 30, 33
Electro-acupuncture 108
Endorphins 102, 105
Enkephalins 105
Eurhythmy 80
Exercise 31, 32
Exercise-induced
    asthma 37

Flu 30
Food allergies 22
Food intolerance 22
Free radicals 45, 46

GLA 50

Gate control theory 105

Hay Diet 42
Hay fever 19
Herbal tisanes 88
Herbalism 55-62
Histamine 17, 27, 42, 43,
    44
Holism 83
Homoeopathy 63-73
House dust mite 16, 22,
    31, 32
Hydrotherapy 78
Hypoglycaemia 42

Immune function 50
Immune system 17, 18,
    24, 28, 29, 41- 45, 47,
    49, 63, 65, 84
Infusions 59
Inhalers 30, 36, 40
Injected steroids 28
Insulin 42
Integrated treatment 89
Intolerance 42
Iridiology 56

Kirlian photography 101

Law of Similars 64
Laxatives 57
Life force 84
Local steroids 28
Lung infection 30
Lymphatic system 87
Lymphocytes 18

Macronutrients 46
Manipulation 95
Massage therapy 85
Mast cells 18

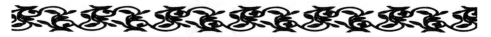

Meridians 105
Micronutrients 46, 47
Milk intolerance 42
Muscular tension 85

Nasal catarrh 87
Nebulisers 25, 36, 37, 38, 39, 40
Nocturnal asthma 32
Nutrition 41-53

Oral steroids 28, 38, 40
Orthodox medicine 25-40
Osteopathy 95-96

Painting therapy 78
Peak flow meter 33, 35
Peak respiratory flow 33
Pollen 15, 16. 22, 27, 29, 31, 44
Pollinosis 16
Pollution 32
Posture 98
Prana 65
Provings 64

Psychosomatic disorder 31
Pulse diagnosis 107

Reductionism 113
Reflexology 99-103
Reflex areas 103
Reflex points 101
Respiratory disorder 87
Respiratory infections 58
Respiratory relaxants 57
Respiratory stimulants 57
Rhythmic massage 78

Sensitisation 18
Skin test 26
Single dose 67
Single remedy 65
Smoking 32
Soft tissue 97
Spasm 58
Speech defect 98
Spinal cord 97
Spinal level 96

Spinhaler 38
Steam inhalation 56
Steroids 24, 28, 29, 30, 32, 37, 55
Stress 86
Succussion 64, 66
Synthesised drugs 55

Thymus gland 44
Tinctures 59
Tisanes 56
Trigger factors 31

Upper respiratory infection 44

Vaccination 44
Vegan diet 41
Vital force 65

Weather 32

Yang 104
Yin 104
Yoga 93

Zone therapy 99

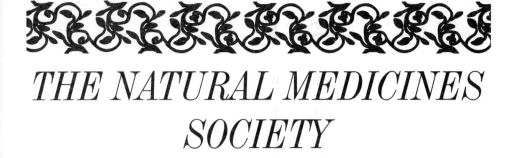

THE NATURAL MEDICINES SOCIETY

The Natural Medicines Society is a registered charity representing the consumer voice for freedom of choice in medicine. The Society needs the support of every individual who uses natural medicines and who is concerned about their continued existence in order to achieve the necessary changes needed to accomplish their wider availability and acceptance within the NHS.

The Society's aims are to improve the standing and practice of natural medicine by encouraging education and research, and by co-operating with the government and the EC on their registration, safety and efficacy. A major drawback in this work has been that none of the Department of Health's licensing bodies has any experts from these systems of medicine sitting on their committees – this has meant that not one of the natural medicines assessed by them has been judged by anyone with an understanding of the therapy's practice. Since the formation of the Society, it has worked towards the establishment of expert representation on the committees appraising these medicines.

To fulfil these aims, the NMS formed the Medicines Advisory Research Committee in February 1988. Known as MARC, its members are doctors, practitioners, pharmacists and other experts in natural medicines. It is the members of MARC who undertake much of the necessary technical and legal work. They have discussed and submitted proposals to the Department of Health's Medicines Control Agency (MCA), on how the EC Directive for Homoeopathic Medicinal Products can be incorporated into the existing UK system, and how medicines outside the orthodox range can be fairly evaluated.

The EC Directive for Homoeopathic Medicinal Products was eventually passed as European law in September 1992, incorporating anthroposophical and biochemic medicines, as well as homoeopathic. With discussions regarding the implementation of

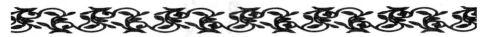

the Homoeopathic Directive now in progress, the MARC's work begins in earnest.

In July 1993, the MCA sent out their consultation paper regarding the implementation of the Directive, which incorporates many of the suggestions submitted by MARC. In it they propose to set up a committee of experts to advise on the registration of homoeopathic, anthroposophic and biochemic medicines. This is a major step forward for the Society, and homoeopathy in general.

With MARC members becoming increasingly involved in the legislative process of the implementation of the Directive, the Natural Medicines Society can now move forward from the short-term aim of protecting the availability of the medicines, to the longer-term aims of promoting and developing their usage and status by instigating and supporting research and education. The NMS has already sponsored some research – it is important to stress here that the Society does not endorse, support or condone animal experimentation – including an expedition to the rain forests in search of medicinal plants, supporting a cancer research project at the Royal London Homoeopathic Hospital and contributing to a methodology Research Fellowship. On the educational side, the Society has published two booklets, with several more planned and has co-sponsored a seminar for doctors and medical students.

The Natural Medicines Society depends upon its membership to continue this unique and important work – please add your support by joining us.

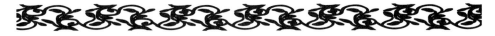

IF YOU ARE NOT ALREADY A MEMBER WHY NOT JOIN THE NATURAL MEDICINES SOCIETY?

Mr/Mrs/Miss/Ms _____ (BLOCK CAPITALS PLEASE) _____

Address _____

_____

Postcode _____ Tel. No. _____

There is no 'fixed' annual membership fee. Please indicate below the amount you wish to pay: minimum £5 (students and unwaged); European countries £15; non-EC £20.

£5 _____ £10 _____ £15 _____

N.B. Pay by Deed of Covenant and/or Direct Debit if you can—please ask for details.

Donations and offers of practical help are also always welcome to aid our fight to return natural medicines to the mainstream of medical practice.

I enclose a donation of £ _____

Please return this form with your remittance (cheques and PO's payable to The Natural Medicines Society), to:

**THE NMS MEMBERSHIP OFFICE,
EDITH LEWIS HOUSE,
ILKESTON,
DERBYS,
DE7 8EJ.**

(Registered charity no.327468)

You will receive your Membership Card, Member's Handbook, Quarterly Newsletter.

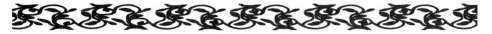

Author Profiles

Hasnain Walji is a writer and freelance journalist specialising in health, nutrition and complementary therapies, with a special interest in dietary supplementation. A contributor to several journals on environmental and Third World consumer issues, he was the founder and editor of *The Vitamin Connection – An International Journal of Nutrition, Health and Fitness,* published in the UK, Canada and Australia, focusing on the link between health and diet. He also launched Healthy Eating, a consumer magazine focusing on the concept of a well-balanced diet, and has written a script for a six-part television series, *The World of Vitamins,* shortly to be produced by a Danish Television company. His latest book, *The Vitamin Guide-Essential Nutrients for Healthy Living,* has just been published, and he is currently involved in developing NutriPlus™: a nutrition database and diet analysis programme for an American software development company.

Dr Andrea Kingston MB ChB, DRCOG, MRCGP, DCH is a Buckinghamshire GP in a five-doctor training practice who has for some years been interested in complementary approaches to healthcare as well as psychiatry and Neuro-linguistic Programming. Hypnotherapy is her major interest, and she has used this technique to help patients throughout the last eight years. As a company doctor to Volkswagen Audi, she contributes regular articles to the company magazine, *Link.* In the past, she has served as a member of the Family Practitioners Committee and as the President of the Milton Keynes Medical Society.

Books by the same authors in the Headway Healthwise series:

- Skin Conditions
- Headaches & Migraine
- Alcoholism, Smoking & Tranquillisers
- Heart Health
- Arthritis & Rheumatism